HOW TO MAKE A PREGNANT WOMAN HAPPY

How to Make a
Pregnant
Woman
Happy

Solving Pregnancy's
Most Common Problems—
Quickly & Effectively

by Uzzi Reiss, M.D. & Yfat M. Reiss

CHRONICLE BOOKS
SAN FRANCISCO

Library of Congress Cataloging-in-Publication Data available.

ISBN: 0-8118-4104-9

Manufactured in Canada.

Design by Pamela Geismar
Typeset in Agfa Rotis Sans Serif with Caravan Borders, ITC
Century and Zapf Dingbats.

Distributed in Canada by Raincoast Books
9050 Shaughnessy Street
Vancouver, British Columbia V6P 6E5

10 9 8 7 6 5 4 3 2 1

Chronicle Books LLC
85 Second Street
San Francisco, California 94105

www.chroniclebooks.com

CONTENTS

How to Use this Book

Got a problem? Simply look up the problem or symptoms in the table of contents or index of this guidebook and go to it.

That's it.

No need to read the book from cover to cover. This guidebook is designed for use by busy men and women on an as-needed basis. The answers to pregnancy's most common problems and questions are organized as follows:

THE PROBLEM:
The name of the problem or symptom.

THE FACTS:
A brief explanation of why this problem occurs in pregnancy.

WHAT YOU CAN DO:
A listing of simple remedies you can use to make your pregnant partner feel better.

WHEN TO GET MORE HELP:
A listing of symptoms that should be referred to her physician.

You now know all you need to make your pregnant woman happy.

1

INTRODUCTION

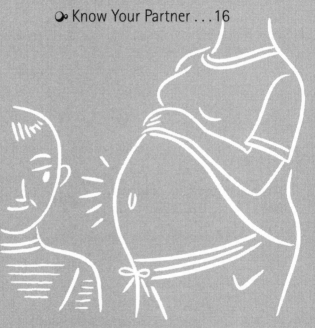

This guidebook is written for men who want answers. If you're looking for an easy way to be helpful to the mother of your child at a time when she needs you most, this book is for you.

How to Make a Pregnant Woman Happy is designed to make it easy for busy men to be attentive fathers-to-be. Simply look up your question or the symptom in the table of contents or the index—go to the section on your topic—and you'll receive a brief explanation of why the problem occurs in pregnancy, a list of easy actions you can take to be helpful and the description of those symptoms that require you to call a physician. *That's it.*

Refer to this guidebook on an as-needed basis. Keep it with you in case your pregnant partner calls you when you're at work or on the go—that way you can always be helpful by telephone.

At every stage of her pregnancy, *How to Make a Pregnant Woman Happy* gives you quick, easy and effective ways to show her that you are engaged and involved, without pages and pages of dense text.

A Special Angle on Natural Home Remedies & Nutrition

In his 30 years as an obstetrician and gynecologist, Dr. Reiss has focused on finding natural and nutritional alternatives to prescription medication. This guidebook arms readers with hundreds of natural home remedies to many of pregnancy's most common problems.

Many of the suggestions recommend a trip to the local health food store over a trip to your pharmacist. Vitamins, minerals and simple changes in diet can go a long way towards making your pregnant partner a happier, healthier and more energetic pregnant woman—and *you* the most helpful partner she can imagine. While Dr. Reiss reasons that we're all better off using these simple, natural remedies whenever possible, this book is not intended to replace regular obstetric care. Always encourage your partner to consult with her physician before taking any of the supplements or using any of the suggestions outlined in this guidebook.

How to Make a Pregnant Woman Happy also focuses on how your words and reassurance can make a difference in her pregnancy—the so-called *mind-body* connection. Never underestimate *your* power to make her feel better.

When to Call Her Physician

Many pregnant women and their partners are reluctant to call their physician when a problem arises—no one wants to be a "high-maintenance" patient.

They've got it all wrong.

Recognize that silence is the *last* thing her physician wants to hear. Physicians aren't psychic; they require a partnership between themselves and an alert patient in order to provide the very best care. More importantly, every physician would rather get a call at 2 A.M.—when something can still be done—than at 9 A.M., when nothing can be done *and* he or she has a waiting room full of patients.

The few hours you wait could make a tremendous difference in the outcome of your child. Be a savvy consumer of health-care services. Identify when your doctor would like to hear from you as follows.

The next time your pregnant partner visits her physician, encourage her to ask:

"What are the symptoms or problems that should cause me to call you at any hour?"

Your chosen physician will describe the conditions that would make him or her *happy* to hear from you. This way you'll never feel uncomfortable about calling—and won't put off getting help for something that requires immediate attention.

Later, when one of you calls the physician regarding a specific problem or concern, always end the conversation by asking:

"What are the symptoms that should cause me to call you again?"

This way you'll always know when to make a follow-up call. And if you or she have forgotten to do this? Call again. Your physician will be glad that you did.

Finally, when the *What You Can Do* sections of this guidebook recommend that you call her physician regarding a specific symptom or test, each section assumes that you and your partner have both decided that a call should be made or that your partner is not able to make the call herself. Realize that some women may be embarrassed or uncomfortable if you contact her physician without her prior knowledge.

Know Your Partner

This guidebook provides a number of suggestions for common problems and symptoms arising during pregnancy. Does this mean that every time she expresses discomfort you should bombard her with 5 or 10 pieces of advice? Not necessarily.

You know your companion best. If she prefers to hear one helpful piece of advice, don't run through the list—this will only frustrate her. On the other hand, if she prefers to be very involved, read the various treatment and prevention options and decide together, or go through each suggestion to determine which appeals to her. Never badger her to confirm that she has followed through. Finally, remember that your most helpful action during her pregnancy may turn out to be no action at all —just a supportive word and a little "sick day" treatment.

2 DIET & DEVELOPMENT

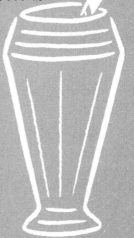

The Problem: **Morning Sickness**

The Facts:

Morning sickness can begin as early as the first days of pregnancy, but generally disappears by the time a woman's pregnancy starts to "show," around the 12th or 16th week of the pregnancy. The most important thing to realize about this "morning" condition is that it isn't limited to morning.

Some women completely escape morning sickness; others experience a weakened version; and some women continue to be plagued by the symptoms of morning sickness straight through their pregnancies.

? How can you tell if your partner is experiencing morning sickness? The first signs are often a complete lack of appetite or loss of appetite after a few bites. But be prepared: These harmless symptoms progress to an uncontrollable need to spit and vomit within minutes.

It is also important to realize that, despite the fact that she may be vomiting, food is the thing that will help her control her illness, and lack of food will make her feel *more* sick. The key lies in determining what foods agree with her pregnant body and how frequently her pregnant body prefers to consume these foods.

What You Can Do:

- Listen to her instincts regarding what "sounds" good. Your partner's body will tell her what is right for her and for the baby.

- Encourage her to eat small amounts of food more frequently. Rather than planning three large meals and a few snacks, suggest that she eat small, balanced meals every two hours. See the *Ideal Pregnancy Diet* section of this guidebook (page 23) for more information.

- Encourage her to eat slowly and see how she feels as she consumes her food, even if she feels very hungry when she begins her meal.

- Suggest that she consume all serving sizes slowly. For example, if she wants an apple, cut it into 10 or 15 smaller pieces and ask her to space out her bites.

- In some cases, women require food more frequently than every two hours. Encourage your partner to listen to her instincts. If she discovers that sipping on a protein smoothie or a mug of soup every 5 to 10 minutes keeps her nausea at bay, then do it. See the *Quick Protein Smoothie* recipe in the appendix of this guidebook (page 199).

- Remember her new favorite pregnancy foods and keep them around.

- Gingerroot is known for naturally alleviating nausea. For this reason it is commonly used by sailors. Get her some raw ginger from the market or under-the-tongue *(sublingual)* drops of ginger extract from your local health food store. Encourage her to carry the ginger drops in her purse.

- Acupressure seasickness bracelets can be helpful if worn all day.

- Vitamins B_5 and B_6, 50 milligrams, three times daily, can also be helpful for warding off morning sickness. Peach tea and two homeopathic remedies called *Ipecac 30X*, 10 to 15 drops as directed, and *Nux Vomica 6X*, 10 to 15 drops as directed, can also be helpful

- Encourage your partner to stay hydrated, even if it means spoon-feeding her water. To cut down on the nausea, add honey or sea salt to her water.

- Small ice cubes are another great way to encourage her to stay hydrated.

Above all, be supportive and don't take offense if it's your cooking that she is vomiting.

When to Get More Help:

If she does not respond to the remedies described above; if her eyes, skin and lips appear dry; if she develops a fever, experiences dizziness and doesn't urinate frequently or has a dark, concentrated urine, contact her physician.

Her physician will likely check her *electrolytes, acid-base balance* and other levels to determine what nutrients she requires.

In severe cases, her physician may opt for solid food replacement to address the fact that she cannot keep food and water down. Many times it is wise to skip the common first treatment of intravenous hydration, because, chances are, your partner's deficiency is not limited to water, sugar and minerals—she may also require protein and fats.

For this, her doctor will prescribe nutrition in liquid form, delivered through an intravenous line or an *NG tube* inserted into her nose and down to her stomach. Your physician will determine the duration and whether this will be done in the hospital or at home.

The Problem: Sensitivity to Smell

The Facts:

Women enjoy an enhanced sense of smell during pregnancy. Consider this a time-tested biological tool designed to help her keep unsuitable food and environments away from her developing baby. Assume that whatever she doesn't like or doesn't smell right to her is not right for your child. Rather than regarding this sensitivity as an annoyance, this strong protective instinct—honed over thousands of years—should be welcomed and heeded.

What You Can Do:

- Encourage her to use this new sensitivity to the baby's advantage. Ask her to smell everything. If a food or soap doesn't smell right, she should avoid eating that food or using that product. If a room seems too stuffy, open a window or move her to another. Defer to her instinct.

- If all food seems to bother her, encourage her to try foods that are organic or those that have not been sprayed with pesticides.

- Consider taking over the food shopping. Aisles and aisles of food smells can be a difficult—often repulsive—experience for a woman with a heightened sense of smell.

- In general, keep the house well ventilated.

- If your cologne or deodorant bothers her, cease using the fragrance and switch to an unscented grooming product.

When to Get More Help:

If her sense of smell is so profound that she is repulsed by everything, contact her physician for a referral to an allergist.

Encourage your partner to use the blank space below to list the foods she craves and those she can no longer tolerate. Suggest she discuss these foods with her physician:

The Problem: **The Ideal Pregnancy Diet**

The Facts:

Diet during pregnancy should be the best that it has ever been. Despite a superb medical infrastructure and a tremendous amount of money spent per capita on food and medical care, North Americans are no champions of health—in fact, many would argue that we lead the world in obesity and disease!

Pregnancy is the time to get back to the basics of nutrition—in the most primitive sense. After all, what goes into her mouth directly affects both mother and child.

The nutritional guidelines provided below are designed to reduce premature delivery, high blood pressure, slow or no fetal development and diabetes of pregnancy.

What You Can Do:

THE DOS:

◌ Encourage her to eat three meals and three snacks every day. She may believe that she is too busy, too sick or too tired to do this, so help her plan what she will eat at various times in the day.

◌ Ensure that she is prepared by accompanying her to the market, or going for her if she finds that aisles and aisles of food make her feel nauseous.

◌ Read labels. Help her avoid processed foods and foods with color additives and preservatives. Encourage her to rediscover more simple foods and to purchase organic meats, fruits and vegetables. Why? Unprocessed foods do not require your baby's body to expend as much energy on detoxifying them, and therefore ensure a more efficient supply of energy and organ development.

☜ Suggest that she eat three eight-ounce portions of protein and a total of 80 grams of protein per day. Lean meat, fish, poultry, dairy, tofu and protein powders are all good sources. Her physician may require that she increase her consumption of protein.

☜ Encourage her to incorporate well-cooked fresh fish into her protein portions. Fish is high in omega-3 fat, which prevents high blood pressure and premature labor, and contains DHA and EPA, essential for fetal brain development. Studies have indicated that babies whose mothers supplemented their diets with these omega-3 fats enjoy increased IQ levels and more regular sleeping patterns.

☜ When choosing fish, encourage your partner to consume non-farm-raised fish varieties, as farmed fish contains a lower level of the beneficial omega-3 fat than non-farm-raised fish. It is common for waiters and fishmongers to provide customers with this information prior to ordering or buying.

☜ When choosing omega-3 fat supplements, such as those containing DHA and EPA, at your local health food store, choose products that indicate that they contain a low level of mercury.

☜ Suggest that she increase her consumption of vegetables. Consider preparing easy soups and salads to expand the variety of vegetables she consumes. The nutrients provided in vegetables are key components in fetal development and the prevention of disease. See the *Easy Vegetable Soup* recipe in the appendix of this guidebook (page 200).

- Eating fruit is an ideal way of controlling sugar cravings, but should be limited to three servings per day due to the sugar content. Vary the type of fruits eaten.

- Remember that all fruits and vegetables must be washed thoroughly. Consider combining water with grape seed extract for a powerful antibacterial wash that will also help prevent gastrointestinal problems.

- Processed carbohydrates, such as breads, pastas, crackers, rice and rice cakes were not available to early humans, and are therefore not part of a "back to basics" diet. If she cannot live without her breads and pastas, encourage her to choose them wisely. Suggest that she pick whole grain breads, pastas and (brown) rice. Remind her that most cereals are mere sugar-delivery vehicles that provide very little in the way of ideal baby nutrition.

- Encourage her to increase her consumption of "good fats" and decrease her consumption of "bad fats." Suggest that she choose foods sautéed or stir-fried with butter, olive oil and canola oil and limit her consumption of saturated fat, fried foods, margarine, hydrogenated or partially hydrogenated oil and vegetable shortening.

- Nuts and seeds are a great way to consume good fats. Encourage her to eat them dry roasted, rather than oil-coated.

- Fruit smoothies provide far more nutrients than plain fruit juice. Add nuts, milk or protein powder for a more complete meal. See the *Quick Protein Smoothie* recipe in the appendix of this guidebook (page 199).

- Most importantly, ensure that she drinks an ample amount of water—no fewer than 8 to 12 glasses a day.

- **Uncooked meat.** Pregnant women should avoid meat that is not fully cooked or is pink in the middle.

- **Prepared ground meat.** Often ground meat has been produced from the meat of numerous animals, increasing the chance of exposure to disease. If she must have a hamburger, buy a single piece of meat and ask your butcher to grind it.

- **Raw fish** (although realize that women in Japan eat sushi throughout their pregnancies). If she must indulge in sushi, ensure that she eats only the freshest possible fish.

- **Large fish.** Tuna, swordfish, shark and other large fish may contain a high level of mercury that is not ideal for pregnant women.

- **Dairy** (if she did not regularly consume diary prior to her pregnancy). Pregnant women receive enough calcium from the leafy vegetables they consume.

- **Fast foods.** These products are often prepared with the lowest quality ingredients—meats, vegetables and oils that you would reject if you saw them at your supermarket.

- **Hydrogenated or partially hydrogenated oils.** These indirectly promote premature labor. Read food labels carefully to avoid these oils.

- **Deep-fried foods.** Generally, deep-fried foods are fried in the cheapest—and least favorable—oils available. If you fry foods at home, lightly fry them in butter, olive oil or canola oil, rather than vegetable oil and margarine, which *hydrogenate* when cooked.

- **Eggs with hard yokes.** Egg yokes *hydrogenate* when they are cooked straight through.

- **Canned foods.** Food stored in cans absorbs properties from the metal containers that are not ideal for pregnant bodies.

- **Artificial colors or sweeteners.** Read food labels carefully to avoid these additives.

- **Sodas and sugary drinks.** Often, these are simply cocktails of impure water, sugar and additives.

- **Alcohol.** It may be difficult for some women to give up a glass of wine after a long week at work. Help her by skipping your alcoholic beverage when the two of you are together.

- **Caffeine and caffeinated products** (including coffee, tea and hot cocoa). Medical information varies on this topic; some studies indicate that up to three cups of coffee per day make little difference. But remember that beverages are not our only source of caffeine—many of the processed foods we eat also contain caffeine. If she likes the ritual associated with a cup of coffee, encourage her to switch to decaffeinated coffee and noncaffeinated herbal teas. When buying decaffeinated coffee and tea, choose products that indicate that the decaffeinating method was "water process."

- **Store-bought or restaurant desserts.** Desserts that are not homemade are problematic, because they are often produced with *hydrogenated* vegetable oil and margarine. If you're dining out or eating at someone else's home, skip dessert or opt for those made with fruit or pure chocolate.

OTHER TIPS:

- Encourage her to eat slowly. Even if she's famished, suggest that she eat for a few minutes and then take a break. This will make digestion easier on her body.

- Encourage her to smell all foods before she begins eating. Pregnant women develop a highly sensitive sense of smell designed to protect their baby from improperly prepared or stored foods. If the food doesn't smell right, encourage her to opt for something else. She should always trust her instincts.

- Most women are overwhelmed by all that they must consume to keep their growing babies healthy. Become the smoothie- or fruit shake–maker of the household. It only takes five minutes to provide your partner with all of the protein, fruits, vegetables, nuts and seeds she requires for the entire morning. Encourage her to drink slowly. See the *Quick Protein Smoothie* recipe in the appendix of this guidebook (page 199).

- Similarly, become a salad chef or soup expert to ensure that your partner consumes a variety of vegetables. When making salad, ask her to smell a selection of condiments to determine which appeals to her. See the *Easy Vegetable Soup* recipe in the appendix of his guidebook (page 200).

- Finally, because it is so important that she eat what she must in order to feed your growing baby, always defer to your partner regarding when, where and with whom she will eat. When dining with friends, help her by suggesting restaurants that cater to the type of food she can eat. Make it easy for her to make the right food choices.

When to Get More Help:

If your partner cannot keep her food down in the first trimester, if you think she isn't eating enough or if she has an uncontrollable craving for sweets, consult with her physician.

The Problem: **Prenatal Supplements**

The Facts:

The first time your partner visits her
obstetrician, she is likely to return
with prenatal vitamins. For some
women this will be an introduction
to daily vitamin supplements, and
for other women, the prescribed
supplements will be a small fraction
of what they already take.

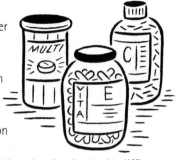

For women who are new to taking vitamins, it may be difficult to swallow several large pills at a time when they cannot
even keep food down in the first trimester. Women who already
take vitamins may be asked to replace their existing supplements
with those prescribed, regardless of whether what they already
take provides their bodies with more nutrition.

Obviously, the ideal situation is for women to see a physician
with an understanding of *nutritional medicine* prior to their
pregnancies. This will allow mother-to-be to begin using nutritional supplements in time for them to be most effective—in the
very first weeks of pregnancy.

What You Can Do:

◌ If your partner is unaccustomed to taking vitamins, and her
prenatal vitamins significantly aggravate her nausea and vomiting, simply skipping her prenatal pills may allow her to eat
more, and thereby receive more nutrients. Consult with her
physician about this option. If she can only take one pill out of
several, encourage her to take her *folic acid* supplement.

◌ Women who are used to taking vitamins and are instructed
to stop taking them may find that their bodies miss the

supplements they used to take. It may be that her physician is unfamiliar with your partner's supplements and may not want to take responsibility for their effect on the pregnancy. Help your partner by consulting a physician—ideally an obstetrician or gynecologist—with experience in nutritional medicine in pregnancy. You'll find that her physician will be happy to allow your partner to proceed with her usual supplement program once he or she receives a recommendation from a physician in the field. In general, only a few common supplements *must* be reduced during pregnancy, including vitamin A (no more than 5000 units), vitamin D (no more than 400 units) and iodine (no more than 0.025 milligrams).

○ It is likely that this will not be your partner's only pregnancy, and that the next pregnancy will be more planned than the first. As such, now is the time to promise yourselves that at least three months prior to your next conception attempt your partner will consult with a physician who has an understanding of nutritional medicine. He or she will evaluate your partner's nutritional and hormonal needs in preparation for her next pregnancy. This opportunity is what every nutritionally oriented physician strives for.

When to Get More Help:

If the supplements provided by her physician cause side effects or if your partner is directed to stop taking supplements that provide her with benefits, seek out a second opinion from a OB-GYN or other physician with an understanding of nutritional medicine.

The Problem: **"Normal" Pregnancy Weight Gain**

(Also see the *Slow Baby Growth* [page 148], *Fast Baby Growth & Large Babies* [page 151] and *"Normal" Pregnancy Growth Rate* [page 35] sections of this guidebook.)

The Facts:

Although women must eat better quality food more consistently during their pregnancy, it is not true that they must "eat for two." This common misconception often leads pregnant women to quickly put on unnecessary weight that is very difficult to shed after the birth of their child. This "pregnancy splurge" can also result in weight gain for the pregnant woman's partner— sometimes referred to as a "sympathy pregnancy." None of this is necessary for the growth of a healthy child.

Extensive weight gain can cause complications. The larger your partner becomes during pregnancy, the clumsier and less active she is likely to be. Neither condition is ideal. Additionally, the more excess weight your partner gains, the statistically larger the baby may grow—which may increase the chances for complications during your partner's labor.

How much and how quickly should your partner gain? Many people assume that women begin consistently gaining weight from the day they conceive. This is not the case:

FIRST TRIMESTER: The growing baby does not add to your partner's weight in the first trimester. In fact, about a quarter of all women lose weight during this period of time. Of those women who put on a small amount of weight (i.e., approximately 5 pounds), the weight is the result of growing breast size, the growth of the uterus, the development of the placenta and the amniotic fluid and the increase of overall blood volume in the mother's body. Absent other conditions, women should not gain more than 10 pounds during the first trimester of pregnancy.

! On the other hand, when women undergo the grueling *hormone induction* cycle associated with many fertility treatments, including in-vitro fertilization, hormones associated with this treatment can visibly increase your partner's weight before she even begins gaining pregnancy weight.

SECOND AND THIRD TRIMESTERS: After the 24th week, or in the beginning of the sixth month, the baby begins to add weight to your partner's frame—but only about half a pound per week. Another half pound of baby-related weight gain per week should also be expected. This consistent level of a total of 1 pound of weight gain per week should be maintained through-out the pregnancy. Gaining more or less than this average should cause her physician to take a closer look at the growth of the baby.

? Why is she showing so much or so little? Your partner's body type has a great deal to do with how "pregnant" she will look during her second and third trimesters. For example, women who are tall and thin may show very little evidence of pregnancy as late as the sixth month. On the other hand, shorter, more voluptuous women, who were at their ideal weight prior to their pregnancies, will look significantly more pregnant despite having put on the same amount of weight as taller women. This is normal.

What You Can Do:

Overeating is far more common than undereating. For this reason, encourage your partner to avoid the "pregnancy splurge." This phenomenon is not good for her, for the baby or for you.

➤ If you didn't do the family shopping before, offer to help out in getting and preparing the family meals. This way you can par-ticipate in choosing what foods come into the house—and what foods are ultimately fed to your baby. Try to purchase raw, fresh foods over processed products. Read labels. Skip those items with sugar or processed carbohydrates that have "empty calories." These foods will not satisfy your partner's hunger or provide your baby with ideal building blocks for brain and body, but they will definitely add to your and your partner's weight.

- Encourage your partner to eat many small meals, rather than three large ones. Many scheduled meals will reduce her desire for snack food.

- Control your own calorie splurges while with your partner. If you must have an indulgent snack or meal, do it when she's not around. Take your partner's pregnancy as an opportunity to clean up your own nutritional act.

- If she turns to you with a pregnancy craving, try to accommodate that craving with a moderate serving or a healthful alternative. Often cravings for sweets can be satisfied with a smoothie, some juice, or even a serving of carrot sticks. A fast-food hamburger can be replaced with a leaner homemade turkey burger and baked "French fries."

- Recognize that your partner's cravings are often the result of a need for a specific nutrient. If she craves a hamburger, it may mean that she requires protein. If she craves pickles, it may mean that her body lacks salt or other minerals. If she craves ice cream, her body may require sugar, protein and fat. Think about this before running off for pickles and ice cream, and consider substituting a healthier alternative.

- Many people eat when they are bored. When your partner asks for a snack between her many meals, invite her out for a slow, romantic walk. This is another great way to increase her activity level and maintain her ideal pregnancy weight.

? What if she insists on eating poorly? If you believe your partner is eating poorly, address the matter openly. Speak to her about the labor complications associated with having a larger baby, about the added clumsiness and the diminished activity level in larger pregnant women. This avoids having to address how the additional weight is changing the way her body looks (and whether you still find her attractive—a sensitive topic), and focuses on medical concerns.

☞ Even in cases when early weight gain is attributed to fertility treatments and hormone injections, you can still encourage your partner to maintain a healthy weight throughout her pregnancy by jointly maintaining healthful pre-pregnancy and pregnancy eating habits.

When to Get More Help:

If you find that your partner is gaining more than 1 pound per week in the beginning of her pregnancy, discuss existing eating habits and ideal pregnancy nutrition with her physician. Your family's usual diet may be inappropriate for pregnancy, and the earlier you correct this, the better.

On the other hand, if you see your partner losing weight or failing to gain weight after the 24th week of pregnancy, be sure to bring this to the attention of her physician.

The Problem: **"Normal" Pregnancy Growth Rate**

(Also see the *Slow Baby Growth* [page 148] and *Fast Baby Growth & Large Babies* [page 151] sections of this guidebook.)

The Facts:

How can you tell whether your baby's size is "on track" throughout the pregnancy? Physicians measure fetal growth rate in *weight,* not length. Approximate fetal length is included below to give you a better idea of the baby's real-world progress:

FIRST TRIMESTER: In the month following conception, your baby will go from a tiny fertilized egg to a .014 inch *embryo*. By the 13th week, the embryo has grown to a 2½-inch *fetus.* Unfortunately, none of this growth is visible to the eye and very little is apparent to the touch.

SECOND TRIMESTER: Between the 13th and 16th week, the pregnancy will "pop" out around the area of the lower pelvis—suddenly the "size" of the pregnancy is apparent. Realize, of course, that the size of your partner's belly does not accurately represent the size of the baby. Your baby will grow to a length of approximately 6½ inches by the 20th week, and nearly 9 inches by the end of the 25th week.

THIRD TRIMESTER: The last third of the pregnancy is when the growth of the pregnancy and the baby will be most apparent to the outside world. Between the 24th and 40th weeks, the line between your partner's pubic bone and the highest point of her belly should increase approximately one centimeter (i.e., a little less than half an inch) per week.

During this period of time, your developing baby will begin growing and gaining weight much more rapidly. Whereas the baby began the 28th week at approximately 9 inches and more than two pounds, he or she will grow nearly 12 inches and gain six or seven pounds by the end of the 40th week.

! Regardless of what's developing on the *inside,* how large
or small your baby looks from the *outside* will be largely
determined by your partner's body type. For example,
women who are short, voluptuous or overweight generally
look like they are carrying a larger baby. On the other
hand, the bodies of women who are taller and thinner give
the impression of a smaller baby. Women carrying multiples (i.e., twins, triplets, etc.) generally look larger, and
all babies look larger when their mother's bladder is full.
The point is, not all babies that appear small are small,
and not all babies that appear big are big.

What You Can Do:

Because the proper rate of your baby's growth is directly related
to his or her well-being, your assistance in monitoring this
growth is crucial. Your participation and vigilance are especially
important in the second trimester, when essential development
occurs weekly and your partner's doctor appointments are
spaced a month apart. For more information on monitoring your
baby's well-being, see the *Monitoring "Normal" Baby Movements*
section of this guidebook (page 142).

◌ Whenever possible, accompany your partner to her doctor's
   appointments. Alternatively, accompany her on a day when
   she will be monitored by *ultrasound.* This will give you more
   concrete information about how the pregnancy is developing.

◌ Make a habit of touching your partner's belly. Feel the baby
   and the pregnancy environment. Does it seem bigger, smaller
   or the same? Helping your partner do this will make it more
   likely that the two of you will make note of any slowing in
   growth rate.

When to Get More Help:

If you believe the baby's growth rate has slowed or stopped, contact your partner's physician. An ultrasound will confirm actual growth rate and will either alleviate your concerns or give her physician the early detection he or she requires.

The Problem: **Breast Tenderness & Breast Enlargement**

The Facts:

Believe it or not, pregnancy is a *dream come true* for breasts. After all, procreation is the reason that women have breasts. Despite the fact that they will only be used once the baby is born, your partner's breasts begin to grow and may become sore from the very beginning of the pregnancy.

What You Can Do:

Often the reasons for breast tenderness and pain are the tight underwire bras and antiperspirants that women wear. Bras obstruct *lymphatic* blood flow, and antiperspirants prevent perspiration. In fact, sometimes bras are so tight that they may cut off the blood flow to the breast area. If your partner experiences breast pain, consider the following:

- Encourage her to go without a bra, or if that is not possible, to wear a *loose,* soft bra or sports bra that does not put pressure on the breasts or the area around the breasts. If she hesitates, tell her you'd like to take her out and buy her a few bras that meet the specifications described above. Tell her she looks beautiful in them.

- Suggest that she switch from antiperspirant to deodorant or her favorite perfume; then buy her some.

- If your partner experiences breast pain because she is retaining water, draw her a *warm* bath. Bath water should not exceed 98 degrees Fahrenheit. Exposure to bath water heated *above* 98 degrees Fahrenheit may increase the rate of birth defects and, in advanced pregnancy, may lead to premature contractions and delivery. Help her climb in and immerse herself up to her neck. Keep her company or stay close by, as she is likely to require a bathroom trip every 15 to 20 minutes, and will need your help for a safe exit and reimmersion. Soaking in water is a great way to move retained water from unwanted areas to areas beneficial to the baby—like the amniotic fluid.

∞ Breast tenderness can also be alleviated by massage. Offer to massage her breasts using the same lotion or paste used to prevent stretch marks. Avoid rubbing this lotion on the nipples, as it could block future milk delivery.

When to Get More Help:

Rarely, breast tenderness is associated with an infection. If your partner develops a red, tender and hot area above the nipples, call her physician.

If your partner feels pain in only one breast, pain that becomes worse when she inhales or pain associated with short-ness of breath or a cough, call her physician. It is likely that the problem lies in her chest, rather than her breasts.

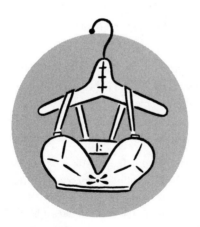

The Problem: **Unresponsive or Inverted Nipples**

The Facts:

The breast is the food delivery vehicle for your baby. As such, the nipple must be ready to deliver when the baby arrives. Inverted nipples, or nipples that do not rise and harden when stimulated by touch, should be brought to the attention of your partner's physician and receive "treatment" by a lactation specialist referred by her physician, your chosen hospital or a friend.

What You Can Do:

◑ If your partner has inverted nipples, ask her to bring this up with her physician.

◑ If her nipples are small and flat, test them to see if they require further attention by stimulating the nipples. Ideally, the nipples should respond by hardening and rising above the surface of the breast. If the nipples do not respond, bring this condition to your partner's attention and request a referral for a lactation specialist.

◑ A suckling baby can be very hard on nipples that had previously only been caressed and lightly fondled. Help your partner's nipples become accustomed to the work ahead of them by encouraging her to wear a T-shirt without a bra. The constant friction will toughen the skin on the nipples.

◑ Alternatively, take a *warm* (not hot) wet hand towel and lightly brush the nipples for a minute every few days. Don't overdo it.

? Does breast size affect the ability to breast feed? Nearly uniformly, the size of the breast has no correlation to milk production. In fact, women with size AA cup breasts can feed a baby with the same success as a woman with size DD cup breasts!

When to Get More Help:

If your partner's nipples are inverted or do not respond, seek the help of a lactation specialist through her physician, the hospital maternity ward or by referral of a friend. Lactation specialists should be consulted several months prior to the arrival of the baby.

3 MOODS & MIND-SET

The Problem: **Mood Swings**

The Facts:

Pregnancy is a virtual symphony of mood swings related to any number of internal conditions, including drastic changes in sugar levels, changes in blood flow, hormone fluctuations and electrolyte and water changes in the body. Focusing on the exact cause of each mood swing is often less important than recognizing that each of your partner's moods is the result of a biochemical change in her body that is real and that *she cannot easily control.* Imagine having to deal with this at work!

What You Can Do:

- Try to help her understand that her mood swings are a natural part of the process. Don't allow bad moods to become opportunities for dwelling on self-doubt. Reassure her of her worth and remind her that her bad mood will pass.

- Don't allow mood swings to create arguments. Be as patient as you would want her to be during your most intense weeks at work. Thank your good luck that you are on the observing end of the mood swing. Transfer this gratitude to additional patience and uncritical attention. Have faith that inside the angry or crying woman before you is your *real* partner, frustrated and not believing the words coming out of her mouth.

- Often mood swings are attributed to other non-pregnancy-related needs. For example, what may seem like a mood swing may simply be a need for rest and a quiet moment. Give her that time and be understanding.

- Finally, recognize that pregnant women can be more sensitive to criticism. If she seems angry, ask yourself whether something you said could have been misunderstood. Her silence may be a product of hurt feelings that she doesn't want to share because she feels that she is *already* complaining too much. Take a deep breath, embrace her and encourage her to confide in you. Most of the time you'll find that the matter can be easily cleared up. If you think about it, this phenomenon isn't exclusive to pregnancy; misunderstandings occur all the time! But in pregnancy, try to give your communication the moments it deserves to strengthen the bond between you.

- Make sure she's well hydrated. Pregnant women should consume between 8 to 12 glasses of water per day.

- Make sure she's snacking every few hours to avoid low blood sugar, or *hypoglycemia*. For more suggestions on this topic, see the *Low Blood Sugar or Hypoglycemia* section of this guidebook (page 157).

- Visit your local health food store for raspberry leaf tea or a fast-absorbing form of *magnesium*, such as *magnesium glycinate, magnesium gluconate, magnesium aspartate* or *magnesium citrate*. Use as directed. These remedies can help calm your partner when she is frustrated. To lift her mood, look for *peppermint leaf tea* or 25 to 50 milligrams of B complex vitamin daily.

When to Get More Help:

If you find that your partner is crying a great deal, or seems quiet, withdrawn and unresponsive, she may be experiencing depression. See the *Depression in Pregnancy* section of this guidebook (page 69) and consult her physician for assistance.

The Problem: **Mental Fogginess & Forgetfulness**

The Facts:

Forgetfulness during pregnancy is commonly reported, but not well-researched.

Physicians often attribute this condition to the extreme fatigue experienced by a majority of pregnant women. Most women overexert themselves during pregnancy. Between new physical discomforts, work in and outside of the home and other commitments, who wouldn't be tired and forgetful?

Another common culprit is dehydration. Women perspire more during pregnancy, and are often reluctant to resupply their bodies in order to avoid numerous trips to the bathroom.

Forgetfulness may also be caused by a natural drop in blood pressure, a condition that peaks between the 20th and 28th weeks of the pregnancy.

Finally, because the body produces more insulin during pregnancy, your partner's blood sugar levels can drop throughout the day. Low blood sugar, or *hypoglycemia,* is a common cause of mental fogginess and may also be accompanied by dizziness and sweating.

What You Can Do:

- Encourage your partner to nap when she needs to. Even a short nap after work can refresh her mind.

- Suggest that she drink between 8 to 12 glasses of water per day.

- Unless specifically restricted by her obstetrician, help her combat low blood pressure and related forgetfulness by encouraging her to add sea salt to her food or water. Most pregnant women are sodium and potassium deficient.

- If she experiences dizziness when she gets up or changes position, if she perspires and cannot concentrate, she may have low blood sugar, or *hypoglycemia.* To remedy this, encourage her to decrease her intake of carbohydrates, starches and sugar and consume more protein, more often. Simply eating a breakfast of orange juice ("flavored sugar water") and toast ("unfavorable carbohydrates") practically ensures that she will feel hypoglycemic by 10 A.M.

- If she experiences dizziness when she gets up, encourage her to take her time, rising slowly and deliberately. Suggest that she lie down and rest when needed. These simple precautions can help avoid a fall that could injure your partner and the baby.

- If she feels dizzy or lightheaded, suggest that she avoid showering or entering a humid bathroom until she feels better, as the heat and steam will make her more lightheaded and prone to falling.

- Be understanding if she is unable to remember details or required tasks. Even without a tendency to forget, pregnancy can be a mentally and physiologically overwhelming process.

When to Get More Help:

If she is making efforts to be well rested and well hydrated and is controlling her blood pressure and sugar levels, but continues to feel foggy and forgetful, consult her physician.

If your partner falls *after* the first trimester, contact her physician with information about how, when and where she fell to determine whether she requires medical attention. Falling in the first trimester is not likely to affect the pregnancy because the fetus is protected by your partner's pelvis at this early stage.

Contact her physician any time your partner feels dizziness that is also accompanied by shortness of breath, headache, blurred vision or heart palpitations.

The Problem: **Headache & Migraine**

The Facts:

Headaches in the first and second trimester are common. Why? Imagine you are perfectly healthy, but wake up one day with nausea, hemorrhoids, indigestion, fatigue, an inability to move quickly and clumsiness when you do move. After a whole day of discomfort, don't you think *you'd* develop a headache, too?

What You Can Do:

Although she may have relied on over-the-counter headache medications prior to her pregnancy, resist the urge to tell her to "pop a pill." Aspirin, *ibuprofen* (commonly known as Advil) and *acetaminophen* (commonly marketed as Tylenol), should not be used unless her physician recommends, as they can affect your partner's liver and the baby's heart and liver. Instead, try a few of the following home remedies:

☞ Apply a cold towel to her forehead.

☞ Take her hands in yours and massage the soft tissue points where her thumb and forefinger meet. Massage clockwise and then counterclockwise for two to three minutes each.

☞ Ask your partner to lie down. Massage her forehead in a circular motion, in between her eyes, where her nose begins. Massage clockwise and then counterclockwise. Then massage her two skull bones, the protruding parts of her forehead, just above her eyes. Finally, massage the crown of her head—where a baby's "soft spot" would be. You'll find that simply taking the time to touch her and be sympathetic will do as much for relieving her headache as the actual massage.

☞ Acupuncture, homeopathy and chiropractic manipulations have been known to be effective for headaches as well.

○ Help her to reduce and avoid daily stress. Things she previously did without effort are now complicated by a myriad of physical problems. Try to lend a sympathetic ear and, when possible, be a problem solver. No obvious way to solve her immediate problem? Suggest a slow walk hand-in-hand and a good talk. Sometimes simply listening is problem solving enough.

○ Skipping meals or not eating frequently enough can cause headaches. Encourage her to eat regularly and keep healthful snacks with her for the hours in between her meals. See the *Ideal Pregnancy Diet* section (page 23) for snack suggestions.

○ Some pregnancy headaches are related to low *thyroid* hormone levels. Taking steps to balance her thyroid will alleviate headaches of this nature. See the *Low Thyroid Levels* section (page 162) for more information on testing and treatment.

○ Supplementing *magnesium* can also help with headaches. Look for *magnesium glycinate, magnesium gluconate, magnesium citrate, magnesium aspartate* or another fast-absorbing magnesium at your local health food store. Encourage her to take the suggested dosage and slowly increase the dosage every few days. Reduce her dosage if she feels fatigued, if her muscles feel weak or at the onset of diarrhea.

When to Get More Help:

Although rare, headaches during pregnancy may be an early indication of neurological problems in the mother. Initial headaches in this period should be reported to her physician, who will determine whether further evaluation is necessary.

Headaches in the late second trimester and third trimester should always be reported to rule out complications associated with high blood pressure.

The Problem: **Insomnia**

(Also see the *Frequent Urination* section
of this guidebook [page 129].)

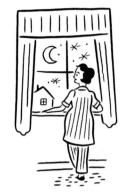

The Facts:

Insomnia in late pregnancy is caused by a
combination of:

- ❯ general discomfort,

- ❯ difficulty in finding a comfortable sleeping position,

- ❯ the baby's pressure on the bladder requiring frequent
  urination, and

- ❯ the body's natural tendency to disrupt sleep in late
  pregnancy, in an attempt to prepare your partner for
  her baby's two-hour feeding cycles.

! Pregnant women should always lie on their sides, rather
than on their backs, to ensure maximum blood flow to the
baby.

What You Can Do:

HELP HER GET TO SLEEP:

❧ At bedtime, turn off the lights and the television.

❧ If your partner is having trouble sleeping, suggest a turkey
dinner or a glass of milk. *Tryptophan,* the amino acid found in
milk and turkey, has been found to be an extremely effective
sleep aid. Avoid chocolate milk and cocoa, as these beverages
contain caffeine. Alternatively, visit your health food store for a
tryptophan supplement called *5 hydroxy tryptophan.* Suggest
she take 50 to 150 milligrams to help her sleep. *5 hydroxy tryptophan* should not be used if your partner is also taking anti-
depressant medication such as *Prozac, Paxil* or *Zoloft* (SSRI).

! Your partner should not take sleeping pills, muscle relaxants or cold medications with antihistamines without the express consent of her physician.

○ For other natural sleep aids, visit your local health food store for *kava kava*, *valerian root* or a fast-absorbing magnesium supplement, such as *magnesium glycinate*, *magnesium gluconate*, *magnesium aspartate* or *magnesium citrate*. Use as directed.

○ In late pregnancy, many women find that they cannot sleep because their babies become active—kicking and turning—when the mother lies down. Conversely, when women move around, their babies are less likely to kick. How can you help your partner get around this contradictory activity? Try music. Many couples find that music lulls their babies to sleep once they arrive. Why not start this "training" *in utero?* Look for tapes and compact discs of relaxing music and use headphones placed on the pregnancy area to quietly "pump" it in. An added bonus: Some couples find that playing music before birth makes their baby more likely to fall asleep to the same music after the delivery.

○ If your partner cannot sleep during the night, encourage her to take naps during the day or early evening when she returns from work. The key is to get sleep whenever possible.

HELP HER GET BACK TO SLEEP:

○ If your partner awakes in the middle of the night and feels the need to urinate, encourage her to get up and empty her bladder.

○ When your partner gets up to use the bathroom, suggest that she keep the hallway and bathroom lights off. This will maintain her body's production of *melatonin*, and help her get back to sleep more quickly.

- To make her nightly bathroom trips more safe, install a small nightlight on her path from the bed to the bathroom.

- As another safety measure, before you turn in each night, take a few minutes to sweep her bed-to-bathroom path of anything she might trip over.

- Further uncomplicate her nightly bathroom trips by suggesting that she sleep on the side of the bed closest to the bathroom.

- When she returns to bed, refrain from engaging her in conversation. Instead, encourage her not to worry, to lie on her side, breathe deeply and relax.

- If your partner cannot sleep due to ongoing concerns about the pregnancy, encourage her to develop a "pregnancy *mantra*." For example, ask her to repeat to herself, *"I'm pregnant; I feel great; my pregnancy is progressing perfectly; and I have a perfect child."* Suggest that she repeat this mantra with eyes closed, between deep breaths, as she visualizes her body sleeping peacefully.

> **!** Some pregnant women wake up at night with heart palpitations, heavy perspiration and a concerned feeling. What causes this? Your mother-to-be may have simply changed position in her sleep and ended up flat on her back. When pregnant women lie flat on their backs, blood flow decreases to the baby *and* to the mother's brain. The decreased blood flow wakes her up so that she changes position. This natural phenomenon is the reason pregnant women need not be concerned about accidentally shifting to a flat position as they sleep.

When to Get More Help:

If your partner cannot sleep for three nights in a row, discuss this condition with her physician.

The Problem: **Her Fears about the Well-Being of the Baby**

The Facts:

There has never been a woman who did not become concerned about the health of her developing child at some point in her pregnancy. Today, these fears are more often based on the *history* of obstetric medicine, rather than the modern reality.

Just 30 years ago, a physician wasn't able to hear the baby's heartbeat until halfway through the pregnancy, and couldn't see the baby until the day of the delivery. For these reasons it was often difficult to confirm that the baby was "normal" until the day that he or she arrived, leading to well-founded anxiety in the mother. After all, a significantly higher percentage of babies were born with birth defects that were not or could not be diagnosed prior to the delivery.

Today, by measuring various hormone levels, it is possible to incrementally confirm the well-being of the pregnancy just one week after your partner's missed period—before there is a trace of the pregnancy in the uterus. Also:

- ❱ By the second week after a missed period, her physician is already able to see the embryo by ultrasound.

- ❱ By the middle of the seventh week of pregnancy—less than two months after your partner's missed period—it is already possible for her physician to monitor the baby's heartbeat by ultrasound.

- ❱ By the tenth or eleventh week, your doctor can also confirm a higher risk of certain chromosomal defects.

All this before her pregnancy is physically apparent!

This provides today's pregnant couple with significantly more reassurance about the well-being of their child. The baby is not unknown; the two of you are able to see him or her and count its fingers long before the delivery. In the event problems arise, her physician may even be capable of correcting them while the baby is still in the uterus. This should help to decrease your partner's concerns about delivering an abnormal child.

> **!** On the other hand, obstetric advancements can some-
> times cause more concern by overdiagnosing. Many times
> ultrasound and other technologies diagnose minor disor-
> ders that may or may not have a significant effect on the
> normal development of the child. As a result, the pregnant
> couple spends several months worrying about a "problem"
> that is quickly dismissed the moment the child is exam-
> ined after delivery.

What You Can Do:

○ Remind your partner of the close watch you, she and her physician are keeping on the baby—a much closer watch than her mother was able to provide.

○ Try to accompany your partner to her doctor's visits. This may be easier to do if you ask her to book early morning, lunchtime or early evening appointments. Between doctor's appoint-ments, remind her of the good progress report given by her physician.

○ As questions or concerns come up, encourage her to write down her questions and to bring this list with her to her next appointment. Ask these questions for her if she fails to.

○ On the other hand, pressing concerns should always be called in to her physician. Note what a "pressing" concern entails; during your part-ner's initial visit, ask the physician to list those symptoms or problems considered to be "pressing."

Remember: Her physician would prefer to hear from you at 2 A.M.—when something can be done—than at 9 A.M. the next day—when it is too late to help.

? What about "older" pregnancies? If your partner is over 30, request that her physician measure her *progesterone* hormone level *weekly* until the eighth week of the pregnancy. Why? Progesterone is one of the chief pregnancy maintenance hormones. In the second month of the pregnancy, the responsibility for producing this hormone shifts from the mother's ovaries to the baby's *placenta*. With "older" mothers, there is a risk that the ovaries may end their progesterone production before the placenta has taken over, requiring weekly monitoring to prevent miscarriage.

◌ Any time your partner's physician has a concern regarding the possibility of a structural defect in the baby, always ask him or her whether a secondary option by a *perinatologist* would be helpful. This is a doctor who has received subspecialty training in reading ultrasound images, and who has the ability to identify and confirm birth defects more easily.

◌ Don't forget that *you* can alleviate many of her fears. Try to make her identify her *specific* concerns. Ask her questions about what—exactly—she thinks is wrong with the baby and what—exactly—will be the negative outcome. Often by carrying fears out to their natural conclusions, they prove themselves to be baseless. Instead, encourage her to visualize that her baby has gifts exactly opposite of the conditions she is concerned about. For example, if she believes her baby will be blind, ask her to visualize that her baby will have the superior eyesight of a jet pilot.

◌ Encourage your partner to create a "pregnancy *mantra*" and use it when she is feeling concerned about the baby. For example, *"I'm pregnant; I feel great; my pregnancy is progressing perfectly; and I have a perfect child."* Suggest that she repeat this *mantra* with eyes closed, between deep breaths.

When to Get More Help:

If you have tried to reassure her, but she continues to focus on her fears, arrange for her physician or other health-care professional to take her, organ by organ, through ultrasound pictures of her baby to show her that the baby is developing properly. This should assuage her fears.

It is common for fears about pregnancy to derive from the bad experiences of family and friends. If this is the case with your partner, contact the maternity unit of the hospital where your partner will deliver, where psychologists, psychiatrists and social workers specialize in working with women who have trauma related to pregnancy.

Finally, if your partner's fears are based on a discovered defect, encourage her to learn more about what can be done for the developing child after the delivery, rather than focusing on her worries. For example, if a physical defect will require surgery, take the opportunity to choose a pediatrician and a surgeon prior to the baby's arrival.

The Problem: **Her Fear about Pain during Labor & Delivery**

The Facts:

Women fear labor and delivery because it is no walk in the park. Fear of this inevitable pain is *real*. Your partner is likely to have heard gruesome stories from family, friends and colleagues, all of whom may have experienced hours of pain *despite* their breathing exercises.

What You Can Do:

To help alleviate her fears about the upcoming pain she may—or may not—endure, try the following:

- Encourage her to avoid stories about pain and agony. Most likely, unless told by her mother or her sister, the stories of strangers will be wholly unrelated to the kind of labor she will have. Learning of yet another horror story will only make her more anxious. On the other hand, did her mother tell her the story of what an easy delivery she had with her? Suggest that your partner focus on *that* story.

- To further quell anxiety, encourage her to visualize an easy birth. For example, ask her to focus on the feeling of when the baby is placed in her arms—even if she delivers by cesarean section (C-section). Focusing on this image will prevent her from spending months fearing what she cannot control.

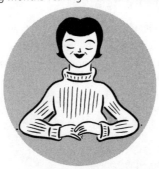

- If her fear of the pain is so great that she would prefer to completely avoid it, find a physician who is willing to order a continuous *epidural* block as soon as she perceives that her pain is too uncomfortable. An epidural is a nerve pain block routinely used in delivery and considered far safer than sedation. If her doctor agrees, make sure that your partner's medical chart reflects this preference and that her physician's entire group (i.e., the alternate doctors who may deliver your partner) and the hospital are able to provide this option.

- Even if you've received an assurance that your medial group and hospital are willing to administer continuous epidural blocks, prepare your partner for the overanxious baby who may not wait for the epidural to be administered. Take birthing classes and make a "Plan B" in which you and your partner will work as a team, whether through breathing exercises, talking or even walking down the halls of the maternity ward. Plan how you will help her focus away from the pain in order to achieve your goal together.

- On the other hand, if your partner plans to deliver without pain assistance, but ends up with an epidural block— that's fine, too. A change in plan midway through the delivery is common and in no way reflects poorly on your partner, her courage, or on her caring for the baby. Labor and delivery are difficult and should be considered a success however she gets through them.

When to Get More Help:

If, in spite of various reassurances, your partner continues to experience extreme anxiety or nightmares, speak to the coordinator of the maternity department where your partner will deliver. He or she will direct you to a staff member who can be of assistance.

The Problem: She Says You're Not Involved in the Pregnancy

The Facts:

Obstetricians commonly hear women complaining that the men in their lives are not involved—or even *interested*—in the developing pregnancy. One common complaint is that men do not accompany the mother-to-be to doctors' appointments.

In reality, you are probably *very* interested in the fact that your partner is carrying your future son or daughter, but may feel—especially at the beginning—that there is very little for you to do. After all, your partner won't even look like she's pregnant until halfway through the process!

Moreover, for many men, competitive pressures at work prevent them from leaving for large portions of the day—essentially 15 half days in seven months—in order to spend 45 minutes in the waiting room and 15 minutes with the doctor. This is especially true when the mother-to-be is also missing work for this purpose. Many men reason that, with new financial responsibilities on the horizon, this is the absolute worst time to look unproductive at work.

The fact is, most obstetricians will tell you that being involved in the pregnancy has very little to do with whether you physically appear at her appointments; many fathers meet their obstetricians for the first time in the delivery room. On the other hand, some of the *least* involved partners show up at *every* appointment.

What matters most is how *she* feels about those efforts that you *can* make to show interest in the pregnancy, regardless of whether you ever set foot into her doctor's office.

What You Can Do:

- If your partner complains about your lack of involvement, despite how frustrated she may sound, encourage her to sit down and calmly pin point exactly what she would like you to do. Turn a nonspecific phrase like "you're not involved" into a specific request that you can act on.

- If her specific request conflicts with other responsibilities—for example, if your job will not allow you to join her for appointments—explain why you feel that your focus on work or some other commitment provides benefits to you all, as a *family*.

- If you cannot accompany your partner to her appointments, become involved from afar. Make note of when her appointments are and discuss the upcoming appointment prior to her visit. If questions have come up since the last time she saw her physician, make note of them and remind her of what she'd planned to ask. If she feels uncomfortable with certain questions, write her physician a short note or ask her to call you while she is in with the physician.

- Ask her to call you as soon as she leaves her doctor's office or call her yourself. Be inquisitive: ask her how the appointment went and what new information she received.

- When you return home on the day of her appointment, continue your conversation about the appointment. Remember, there will be new information about the developing baby every time she returns; show interest in this.

- See the *Monitoring "Normal" Baby Movements* section of this guidebook (page 142) for information about helping her monitor the baby's movements in a "Kick Journal." Help her with this monitoring by placing your hands where she indicates the baby is moving and putting your ear against her belly.

- Show interest in what she eats—but don't question every food choice.

- Show interest in how much and how often she exercises. Encourage her to maintain her activity level by inviting her out for slow, romantic evening walks.

- Show interest in her concerns about the pregnancy and upcoming delivery. See the *Her Fears about the Well-Being of the Baby* (page 53) and *Her Fears about Pain during Labor & Delivery* (page 57) sections of this guidebook for more information.

- Recognize that in this time—more than ever—she is looking for you to fill the role of *protector*. Help her feel that someone is helping her—watching out for her and her well-being—during this vulnerable and exciting time. Consider this your moment to shine as her *hero*. Be interested and make obvious, even *exaggerated* attempts to show your interest in her, her health and the baby. She may regard your dramatic demonstrations as odd, but inside, she'll consider herself the luckiest woman she knows.

- Encourage your partner to maintain (or begin!) an exercise and stretching program during her pregnancy. Studies indicate that more active and limber women tend to recover from the physical stress of labor more quickly.

When to Get More Help:

If you and your partner cannot reconcile the fact that she thinks you should be missing work for certain events or provide other assistance that you feel you cannot, seek the help of a third party —a mediator, clergy person or a friend—*before* your baby arrives. Do not keep any issue of this nature unresolved, as it may affect your ability to function as a team in the future. After all, who needs to begin a marathon with a sprained ankle?

The Problem: **You Feel Disconnected from the Pregnancy**

The Facts:

Many men have a hard time "connecting" with their partner's pregnancy in the first and second trimester. It's not a lack of interest in their future son or daughter, it's just that there seems to be very little a man can do in those first few months!

Why is this?

While women may begin to feel like mothers—emotionally and physically—as soon as they learn that they are pregnant, men often take a longer time to adjust to—or even be *conscious* of—their new role. Of course, men will be happy and overwhelmed by what they perceive to be their new commitments, but because their information about the baby will often be received second-hand, and because the pregnancy will not become visually apparent from the outside until it is nearly *half* over, some men may "forget" that their partners are pregnant for days at a time! In short, all of this contributes to men feeling that they have very little to do with the pregnancy process.

What You Can Do:

◌ Skim through some of the sections in this guidebook. It's designed to show you how essential you are to the positive outcome of your partner's pregnancy. Ever feel that your professional efforts don't really affect the world one way or the other? By contrast, what you do during the pregnancy *directly* affects your child's future and how your partner regards the experience. Consider this your big chance to be a *hero*.

◌ Try to learn more about the various stages of early pregnancy. This will make your baby's development in the first trimester more real for you. See the *Ideal Baby Growth Chart* in the appendix of this guidebook (page 188).

- If your work schedule permits, make an effort to visit the obstetrician with her—especially on an ultrasound day. Often early morning or evening appointments are available.

- If you cannot accompany your partner to her appointments, be sure to follow up with her about what happened at the appointment and what she learned about the development of the baby.

- Make a habit of asking about her physical condition or concerns about the baby. You may be concerned about the same thing, which could lead to a productive conversation.

- Make a point of touching her belly when she feels the baby kicking. Help her monitor the baby's movement as described in the *Monitoring "Normal" Baby Movements* section of this guidebook (page 142).

- Help her with food choices, exercise maintenance and choice of personal care products. Recognize that everything she eats, does and uses will affect your future child, so your involvement is important!

When to Get More Help:

Because men receive the majority of their information about their baby's development secondhand, and details can be lost in the translation, there may be a time in the pregnancy when you believe something is not progressing as it should. If you require additional information, don't hesitate to pick up the phone and leave a message for her physician or medical staff. Often, with additional information your concern can be easily alleviated.

The Problem: **Your Fears about Assisting in Labor & Delivery**

The Facts:

In modern labor and delivery, men have been assigned the duty of being their partner's "coaches." This is an entirely new role for men! Long gone are the days of waiting out the labor in another room or at the bar down the street, then handing out cigars when the good news arrives. These days, men are expected to join their mother-to-be in the trenches of delivery!

Despite their enthusiasm about the pregnancy and their strong feelings for the women in their lives, some men have significant reservations about being present during the delivery. Often they feel torn between this modern duty and concerns about what they might see and how this will affect the way they view their sexual partners in the future.

Are you failing her by declining this mission?

What You Can Do:

◐ The truth is, whether or not you choose to fulfill the role of birthing coach has very little to do with how good of a father or partner you will be. *Forcing* yourself to participate—or even *attend*—a delivery makes little sense. You may even get in the way!

◐ On the other hand, realize that the birth of your child is an unusual opportunity. This may be one of the only times in your lives as a couple when *your* presence, *your* words and *your* touch can entirely change the way she experiences a physically and emotionally challenging event. No amount of financial support can replace this. *Your* presence is the one thing that can make a difference. Make her see you as her *hero* and create a lasting bond between you.

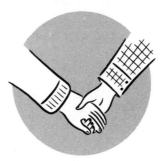

◌ In fact, the men who believe that they are the least prepared for or interested in the delivery often turn out to be the most helpful.

◌ Some men have seen movies of deliveries or have heard "war stories" that make them concerned about the graphic nature of the event. Many men are concerned that witnessing a birth may affect their future sexual desire and ability to perform with their partners. These are legitimate fears that should be respected. However, realize that it is entirely possible to participate in her delivery without *ever* seeing the baby's exit from the birth canal. By simply positioning yourself at her bedside— at her hands and face, and where she would no doubt most like you to be—you can avoid viewing the "graphic" aspects of the delivery. If this is your preference, simply speak to her physician and the nurses assisting the delivery. Many men with these concerns report that when they see their partners' thankful eyes and glowing faces at the moment of delivery— with no graphic elements in view—they are very glad they decided to participate.

When to Get More Help:

If you believe that you cannot participate in the delivery due to squeamishness, travel commitments, or concerns about your ability to provide very active coaching in the event that mother-to-be is committed to a delivery without pain medication or epidural anesthesia, there are alternatives.

Speak to your partner about your concerns and preferences as early as possible. The ninth month is the wrong time to announce that you will not be participating in the delivery.

Traditionally, a mother, other relative or friend served the role of a birthing companion. Speak to your partner about whom she would prefer in your absence. There is also the option of hiring a professional birth coach, or "doula."

Doulas are nonmedical birthing assistants that fill the role generally provided by expectant fathers, family or friends, by helping women breathe, push and focus through the delivery. Many doulas also specialize in a variety of alternative healing methods, including massage, acupressure, aromatherapy and positioning, all of which may assist women in labor.

The great majority of doulas are highly professional, although a few have been known to overstep their roles and training by giving medical opinions or performing pelvic exams. *Neither* of these are appropriate and are beyond the scope of doula services.

If you choose to engage a doula, be sure to communicate what you want her role to be. The doula is not there to take over your birth experience, but to facilitate what you want as a couple and as a family. Doula-assisted deliveries can be wonderful, but physicians often conclude that the expectant father has missed out on a wonderful opportunity.

The Problem: **Your Concerns about Being Replaced by the Baby**

The Facts:

It is common for men to develop concerns that their partners will become so devoted to the baby as to be neglectful of their "number one guy."

In fact, it *is* common for women to become so involved with an infant, that they lose sight of the need to maintain a special connection with their partners.

Is it "all about the baby" from here on out? It doesn't have to be.

What You Can Do:

Ensuring that you and your partner maintain an adult relationship that is separate from your role as parents depends largely on your existing dynamic and on your ability to verbalize your needs for her companionship:

- Talk about your concerns during the pregnancy—before you are both overwhelmed by the challenge of having a new baby in the house. Stress the importance of continuing an ongoing romance once the baby arrives. After all, a good marriage is the best thing you can give to your child.

- After the baby arrives, recognize that your partner will require an adjustment period. The arrival of the baby will require her to recover physically and then learn to balance the needs of the baby with all of her existing responsibilities. She will have to "find" more time than she's ever had before. As a result, she is likely to steal time away from herself and from the time she once had with you. Give her a month or two to become adjusted to this change.

- If, after the first few months, you begin to feel that the romance has waned, don't wait! Express this concern and allow her to express her's. After all, she may be too overwhelmed by the care of a new baby—and all of her existing responsibilities—to read between the lines.

- Follow up your conversation by actively engaging in romantic activities. Call her from work—speak to her in the same tone of voice you used when first courting her. Leave her notes. Come home with gifts. Plan romantic evenings or weekend days by arranging for childcare. Don't wait for romance to happen, *make* it happen—just as you did when you were first dating.

- Remember, the arrival of a child should not destroy the dynamic that brought you together. Healthy children must ultimately adapt themselves to *your* lifestyle. Perhaps she has lost sight of this and needs a reminder.

- When in doubt, don't stay late at work or meet up with the guys. Go home and embrace the woman you chose. Recognize that you have a right to express your basic needs as well. After all, this is the reason you chose to be together and start a family in the first place.

When to Get More Help:

If your partner fails to respond to your concerns, despite implementation of the suggestions above, consider seeking the assistance of a family counselor. Everyone responds to a different wake up call; perhaps speaking to an outside party will be just what she needs.

The Problem: **Depression in Pregnancy**

The Facts:

The sharp change in customary lifestyle, including dress, work, diet, personal grooming, leisure time, intimate contact and the curtailed use of recreational tobacco and alcohol, all affect the mood of the pregnant woman. After all, if you were restricted from doing so many of the things you enjoy, wouldn't it depress you? Depression during pregnancy is caused by several factors:

- The change in body configuration and related changes to self-image.

- The inability to clear one's mind through regular exercise due to morning sickness in early pregnancy.

- Pregnancy-related low blood sugar, or *hypoglycemia,* which causes anxiousness and, in some cases, depression.

- Relative low thyroid condition, or *hypothyroidism,* which causes fatigue and, in some causes, depression.

- Concerns about the well-being of the baby.

- In some cases, pregnancy is regarded as a solution to a variety of personal problems. Depression may develop as the pregnancy progresses and the underlying problems fail to disappear.

What You Can Do:

As her companion, feel empathy toward the pregnant woman—she's dealing with many confusing variables at one time. Recognize that this is the wrong time for casual criticisms or arguments that can be avoided. Avoid critical comments about her changing body, her mood changes or her inability to be as active or perform as many household chores. Let a few things roll off your back every day. You'll thank yourself later—and so will she.

- Be helpful. Be complimentary. Be understanding. Be the first to give in, encourage and participate. Be a take-charge guy during the time she needs you to be. Show her that small problems don't rattle you. Imagine that you're both on a canoe, with you steering and powering the vessel forward from behind. Consider that this is your big chance to show her that you are, indeed, her superhero. The better she feels about herself, the easier *your* daily life will be.

- Remember that a daily kind word and an understanding smile may mean far more than a store-bought gift.

- For concerns about depression caused by *low blood sugar,* see the *Low Blood Sugar* or *Hypoglycemia* sections of this guidebook (page 157).

- For information on helping with pregnancy fears, see the *Her Fears about the Well-Being of the Baby* (page 53) and *Her Fear about Pain during Labor & Delivery* (page 57) sections of this guidebook.

- For concerns about depression caused by fatigue, see the *Fatigue* section of this guidebook (page 72).

When to Get More Help:

If you believe your partner's depression is worsening or not otherwise waning, consult her physician.

4 ACHES & ACTIVITY

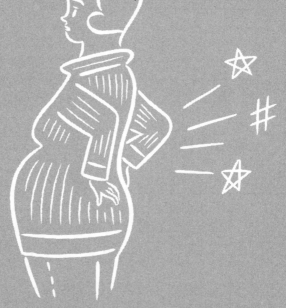

The Problem: **Fatigue**

The Facts:

It would be difficult to find a woman who has not become fatigued in pregnancy. Even those women who seem to breeze through the process eventually feel the burden of extra weight and various other physical discomforts.

For this reason, when pregnant women complain that they feel fatigued, they are generally assured that it is "normal." But can fatigue—and related frustrations and unhappiness—be prevented or minimized? Absolutely. The key is to identify the particular cause of her fatigue and address it.

What causes fatigue in pregnancy?

FIRST TRIMESTER: In the first trimester, fatigue is often caused by a change in blood volume, a deficiency of sodium, potassium and magnesium, low blood sugar, anemia, a low thyroid level and nausea.

SECOND TRIMESTER: In the second trimester, fatigue is most often caused by low blood sugar, sodium and potassium deficiencies, a low thyroid level and anemia.

THIRD TRIMESTER: In the third trimester, new feelings of fatigue are caused by the burden of carrying additional weight, water retention, sleep disruption, an increase in aches and pains, low blood sugar, a low thyroid level and anemia.

What You Can Do:

➤ **Changes in blood volume.** In the first trimester of pregnancy, your partner's body will begin producing a significant amount of additional blood volume within a relatively short period of time. This increases the demand for fluids and often causes dehydration, which leads to fatigue. To avoid this, encourage her to increase her consumption of water. Ideally, she should drink 8 to 12 glasses of water per day.

- **Sodium and potassium deficiencies.** Many of us are concerned with lowering our sodium intake when we should be adding it to our diets. Ask her physician to tests her *electrolyte* and *acid-base balance* to determine what she requires to bring up her readings to an *optimal,* not merely "normal," level. Suggest that she add sea salt to her foods—this supplements both sodium and potassium. Additionally, encourage her to eat more whole fruits and vegetables, either raw or in soups and smoothies. See the *Quick Protein Smoothie* (page 199) and *Easy Vegetable Soup* (page 200) recipes in the appendix of this guidebook.

- **Magnesium deficiency.** Today's foods are often fortified with calcium. In many cases, this creates a calcium-magnesium imbalance when calcium enters the cells and forces magnesium into our bloodstream. The result? An instantaneous feeling of fatigue or sleepiness for several hours. The presence of calcium also destroys the *mitochondria,* the power generators of the body, causing longer-term fatigue. Your mother-to-be can avoid this by supplementing fast-absorbing magnesium, such as *magnesium glycinate, magnesium gluconate, magnesium aspartate* or *magnesium citrate,* available at your local health food store. Use as directed, slowly increasing her dosage every few days. Reduce her dosage if she experiences fatigue, muscle weakness or diarrhea. Additionally, encourage her to watch that she does not consume more calcium than magnesium and eats more whole fruits and vegetables.

- **Low blood sugar or hypoglycemia.** See the *Mental Fogginess & Forgetfulness* section of this guidebook (page 46) for more information.

- **Nausea.** Nausea often prevents women from eating and drinking as much as they should. This mild malnutrition can severely impact your partner's energy level. For more information on preventing nausea in pregnancy, see the *Morning Sickness* section of this guidebook (page 18).

- **Low thyroid level or hypothyroidism.** A low thyroid function can significantly reduce your partner's energy. In pregnancy, even a level that is on the low side of "normal" may not be enough, as thyroid levels may deteriorate in the second and third trimesters. See the *Low Thyroid Levels* section of this guidebook (page 162) for guidelines on thyroid testing.

- **Anemia.** Due to the significant increase in blood volume associated with pregnancy, many women experience a deficiency of iron, folic acid and vitamin B_{12}, also known as anemia. This condition is common in pregnancy and significantly contributes to fatigue. Ask her physician to check her iron levels, not by measuring her *hemoglobin* or *hematocrit* levels (which automatically drop in pregnancy due to the increase in blood levels), but her *true iron, iron reserve* and *iron saturation levels.* Iron should not be supplemented unless her true iron levels are low, as excess iron can increase complications in pregnancy.

  Many iron supplements, including *iron sulfate,* may cause indigestion and constipation. If her physician has prescribed iron supplements, visit your local health food store for other iron supplements that are easier on the gastrointestinal tract. See the *Constipation* section of this guidebook (page 103) for more information.

  Also ask her physician to check her *folic acid* and *vitamin B_{12}* levels. Your partner's vitamin B_{12} and folic acid levels should be optimized to the upper level of "normal" for the duration of her pregnancy. Supplement 1000 micrograms of vitamin B_{12} daily, by way of drops taken under the tongue, available at your local health food store. Alternatively, her physician can provide her with vitamin B_{12} injectables. Supplement one milligram of folic acid daily, also available at your health food store.

- **Additional weight.** As pregnant women put on more weight in the third trimester, they must expend more energy on everyday movement. This exacerbates their fatigue. Help your partner make this last stretch of pregnancy as easy as it can be. Help around the house and with your other children. Encourage her to take frequent breaks and refrain from being more physically active than necessary.

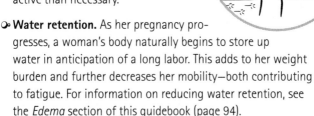

○ **Water retention.** As her pregnancy progresses, a woman's body naturally begins to store up water in anticipation of a long labor. This adds to her weight burden and further decreases her mobility—both contributing to fatigue. For information on reducing water retention, see the *Edema* section of this guidebook (page 94).

○ **Sleep disruption.** In the third trimester of pregnancy, a woman's body begins preparing her for repeated late-night feedings by making it very difficult for her to sleep more than two hours at a time. This cycle of interrupted sleep is likely to increase her fatigue and affect her mood. Encourage her to catch up on her sleep when she can. A short nap in the afternoon or early evening can be very helpful. See the *Insomnia* section of this guidebook (page 51) for more information.

○ **General pregnancy aches and pains.** Finally, realize that any kind of ongoing pain and discomfort is tiring. The more you can do to relieve her back pain, leg cramps, acid reflux and other discomforts, the more energy she'll have and the more her mood will improve. See the sections of this guidebook related to your partner's particular complaint.

When to Get More Help:

See her physician to diagnose low thyroid, anemia and electrolyte imbalance. If, after applying the suggestions described above, your partner continues to experience fatigue, contact her physician for additional help.

The Problem: **Back Pain**

The Facts:

Back pain is common in the second half of pregnancy. The combination of weight gain, loss of the usual center of gravity, decreased activity, mobility and an inability to stretch and straighten out their backs all conspire to create back troubles for pregnant women. Additionally, exacerbation of previous conditions that caused back pain prior to the pregnancy may increase pain during this time.

What You Can Do:

○ Help your partner address back pain as she would have before her pregnancy—with one exception: No pain medication should be taken without the express consent of her physician.

○ Unless otherwise advised by her physician, encourage her to be active throughout her pregnancy. This will ensure that her back is strong for late pregnancy. Pre-pregnancy abdominal workouts can be maintained until the 14th week, and swimming is an excellent low-impact back strengthening exercise in any trimester.

○ Help her stretch out her back as she lies on her side.

○ Encourage her to sleep on her side, with one pillow under her neck and a second pillow between her legs. Lying flat on her back may cut off blood flow to the baby.

> **!** Some back injuries require the use of X-rays and CT scans. Avoid these procedures. MRI procedures are permitted, so long as your partner lies on her side.

○ Help her locate alternatives to back pain medications. Many pregnant women find that acupuncture and chiropractic treatments are helpful. Assist her in seeking out pain specialists, including those physicians trained in *prolotherapy,* a pregnancy-safe treatment wherein a pain trigger point is injected with local anesthesia and concentrated sugar.

! **Pregnant women should not use back support belts designed for weight lifters and moving professionals, as these belts put pressure on the abdomen.**

○• Help her find one of several back straps designed for pregnant women that lift the pregnancy area, giving support to the back and the uterus. Encourage her to wear these straps loosely around her abdomen.

When to Get More Help:

Severe back pain in very early pregnancy, especially when accompanied by abdominal pain, pelvic pain, shoulder pain, vaginal bleeding and faintness, may be a symptom of the rupture of a pregnancy that has developed outside of the uterus. This condition requires the immediate attention of her physician. Otherwise, contact her physician if her back pain is severe, if it radiates into her legs or if she feels numbness in parts of her legs.

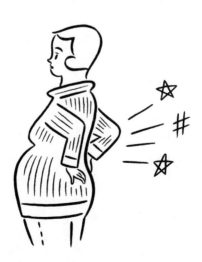

The Problem: **Leg Cramps**

The Facts:

Leg cramps are very common in pregnancy and are most often caused by *magnesium, thyroid* and *electrolyte* deficiencies. In fact, often leg cramping is the first symptom of a thyroid deficiency in adults.

What You Can Do:

- While many physicians commonly prescribe calcium supplements to alleviate leg cramping, this short-term solution has the longer-term disadvantage of depleting the cells of magnesium. By removing what little magnesium the cell has—thereby temporarily flooding the blood with magnesium and soothing the leg cramps—this remedy ultimately magnifies the magnesium shortage and the associated leg cramping. An alternative remedy is as close as your local health food store. Look for *magnesium glycinate, magnesium gluconate, magnesium citrate, magnesium aspartate* or another fast-absorbing magnesium. Encourage her to take the suggested dosage with food, and slowly increase the dosage every few days until her pain decreases. Reduce her dosage if she experiences fatigue, muscle weakness or diarrhea.

- Encourage your partner's physician to test her thyroid level using the *Free T3* and *Free T4* thyroid tests. For more information on proper thyroid testing in pregnancy, see the *Low Thyroid Levels* section of this guidebook (page 162).

- Encourage your partner's physician to test her *electrolyte* levels.

- Suggest that your partner add sea salt to her food. Most pregnant women may be sodium and potassium deficient.

- Often supplementing your partner's diet with 400 to 800 units of vitamin E can be helpful. Look for a high quality vitamin E product at your local health food store.

- Elevate your partner's legs at night with one or two pillows.

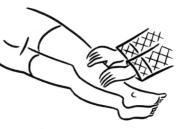

- Try gently massaging your partner's legs along the calf muscles. This can be soothing and preventative.

When to Get More Help:

In rare cases, clot formation in the arteries and inflammation of the veins feel very similar to leg cramps. If your partner's leg cramps continue and she develops a painful, inflamed red line from the ankles up the back of the calf, have your partner's legs examined by a physician.

The Problem: **General Pain**

The Facts:

Pain in pregnancy is a delicate issue. On the one hand, there are many discomforts associated with pregnancy, but on the other hand, pregnant women are just as likely to develop medical problems *not* associated with pregnancy. Moreover, pregnancy can mask symptoms or cause common symptoms to express themselves in unusual locations. For example, appendicitis pain during pregnancy is felt in a different location than when a woman is not pregnant.

The result is that pregnancy may prevent many women from seeking medical help they need and would otherwise obtain. Alternatively, women and their doctors may both assume symptoms or early signs are merely side effects of pregnancy and fail to suspect another condition.

What You Can Do:

↝ If your partner experiences pain that becomes more severe or more frequent despite reassurance from her obstetrician that the ailment has nothing to do with her pregnancy, help her by arranging an appointment with a physician who specializes in the part of the body producing the pain. Have her see an orthopedic surgeon for back pain, a cardiologist for heart palpitations or a neurologist for persistent headaches.

↝ Once she has seen a specialist, recognize that, due to her pregnancy, the diagnosis process may be more complicated. The specialist is likely to avoid certain tests unless her condition becomes life threatening. This is also true of procedure and medication options. Your help can be very valuable in this process. Ensure that your partner does not fall through the cracks—with continuing pain but no available treatment because of her pregnancy. Become her advocate and insist that her physician work with her other doctors to find a creative treatment option.

○∙ If her physicians are unable to identify a problem and have assured her that she is healthy, help her find natural alternatives to traditional treatments or professionals that assist with pain management.

When to Get More Help:

Always consult another physician if she develops symptoms that persist or become worse despite consultation, as these problems may be unrelated to her pregnancy.

The Problem: **Activity & Exercise Restrictions**

The Facts:

Pregnancy is a great incentive to become more healthy. It is the rare woman who picks up bad habits during her pregnancy, as most women take the opportunity to cut out a variety of vices during this time.

Absent contrary physician's advice, pregnancy is also a great time to begin an exercise program, even if she has never been active before. The benefits of this change in routine will be enjoyed by both mother and child in the long term.

FIRST TRIMESTER: Absent aggravated morning sickness, most women find that they can continue with a majority of the activities they enjoyed prior to their pregnancy.

SECOND TRIMESTER: With a few restrictions on activity, the second trimester is a great time to build up cardiovascular fitness—your partner will need the extra lung power as her weight increases.

THIRD TRIMESTER: Cardiovascular activities from the second trimester can be decreased in the third.

A few simple guidelines can help you be your partner's motivator and protector.

What You Can Do:

GENERAL TIPS:

- Women who did not exercise prior to their pregnancy should begin walking, swimming, using a treadmill or riding a stationary bicycle; all *slowly.* If she is not the gym-going type or believes that she does not have time for a workout, invite her for a window-shopping walk around a shopping mall or commercial area.

- Never allow her to become overheated or dehydrated while exercising. Encourage her to rest and rehydrate during any activity.

- Help her recognize that she and the growing baby are competing for the same food. As such, food energy used to exercise is necessarily food energy being diverted away from the baby. For this reason, encourage her to limit her cardiovascular workouts to the lower level of her capacity. She should never get to a point where she is short of breath or unable to speak easily. As a general rule, her active exercise pulse rate should never exceed 135. Encourage your partner to adjust her exercise to her new condition.

- Women who are go-getters may become overzealous about exercise during their pregnancy. This is particularly true for fitness professionals and professional athletes, who should discuss their level of activity with their physicians before resuming normal routines. Remember, in pregnancy, even professional athletes experience reduced coordination, balance and stamina, increasing the probability for accidents to occur.

- Realize that dehydration and overexertion put her pregnancy at risk and could lead to premature labor. If she begins to feel dizzy, nauseous or experiences a contraction during any activity, insist that she stop, hydrate herself and rest by lying on her side.

TIPS FOR SPECIFIC ACTIVITIES:

- **Walking.** Romantic walks are a wonderful opportunity for her to be active and for the two of you to spend time together in any trimester of pregnancy. As you walk, encourage her to breathe deeply and rest when required. And who knows; you may begin a healthy habit that will keep you both active long after her delivery.

- **Hiking.** Women in their first trimester may hike as they did prior to their pregnancy. Hiking in the second and third trimesters should be limited to asphalt trails that are not slippery, uneven or remote. Ensure that she is always accompanied.

- **Swimming.** Swimming is the ideal physical activity during any trimester of pregnancy. Water activities are less strenuous on the joints and—for some reason—appear to compete for energy the least with the growing baby. If she tires of swimming, encourage her to walk back and forth in the shallow end of the pool. Swimming at the beach should be limited to strong swimmers, swimming with a partner close to shore and on a day with calm waters.

- **Bicycle riding.** Pregnant women may bike ride as usual in the first trimester, but limit themselves to a stationary bicycle thereafter.

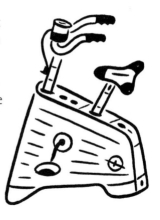

- **Aerobics.** First trimester aerobics classes should be limited to those that do not overexert your partner. In the second and third trimesters, she should avoid classes that involve jumping or stepping up and down, as these may challenge her changing sense of balance.

- **Free weights.** In the first trimester, free weight workouts need not be reduced. When she enters her second trimester, encourage her to reduce the weights she works with, while increasing her repetitions and working them more slowly as she inhales and exhales. Many fitness professionals indicate that this focused approach is more effective for muscle development and maintenance.

Also recognize that, due to a diminished sense of balance during pregnancy and because free weight workouts depend on balance, weight machines may be a safer route during this time. Alternatively, ensure that she always enlists the help of a strong spotter. When lying down for a set, suggest that she to tilt her body slightly to the right or left. Lying flat on her back may cut off blood flow to the baby. Lying on her abdomen is not permitted. Free weight lifting should be limited during the third trimester. For more information, see the *Heavy Lifting & Falling during Pregnancy* section of this guidebook (page 87).

◌ **Stationary bicycle classes.** While stationary bike riding is helpful throughout her pregnancy, the rooms in which cycling classes are held tend to be stuffy and lend themselves to overheating. Encourage her to avoid these classes if she feels her skin becoming hot. Suggest that she peddle at half the rate of the class, wear earplugs to protect her ears and hydrate herself frequently.

◌ **Stretching and yoga.** Stretching and yoga can be a wonderful activity during any trimester of pregnancy. However, due to the presence of the pregnancy hormone *relaxin* (the hormone than relaxes bone joints in order to move the pelvis out for delivery), women are more prone to overextend joints and muscles, leading to increased injury during this time. Encourage your partner to be extra careful with her movements.

Some yoga rooms are heated to enhance flexibility. Pregnant women should avoid rooms heated above 98 degrees.

◌ **Tennis.** Tennis is not restricted in the first trimester. She may continue playing tennis into her second and third trimesters if she limits her game to *completely noncompetitive* play; no jumping for the ball, as this may lead to slipping and falling.

◌ **Sailing.** Sailing and boating are not harmful in the first trimester, but may exacerbate "morning sickness." Due to a decreased sense of balance in pregnancy, always accompany her when she moves about the deck. Take extra care to ensure that she does not lose her balance on slippery surfaces. She should not sail on rough seas during the second and third trimesters.

◑ **Horseback riding.** Riding in the first trimester is fine, but unless she is a professional rider on a horse with no history of being out of control, she should not ride in the second and third trimesters. Realize that even "good" horses can become unpredictable in unpredictable situations.

◑ **Kickboxing.** She should not engage in kickboxing during any trimester of pregnancy.

When to Get More Help:

If your partner would like to engage in an activity not described above, consult her physician.

If she falls, suffers a bodily impact or injures herself while engaging in physical activity, always contact her physician. He or she will determine whether she requires further an evaluation.

The Problem: Heavy Lifting & Falling during Pregnancy

The Facts:

As her pregnancy develops and takes on weight, each woman's center of gravity changes. This change affects her sense of balance and makes her more likely to fall. The weight of an object carried often contributes to a feeling of imbalance. Apart from the usual injuries, falling on the abdomen during pregnancy risks injury to the child and miscarriage. For this reason, it is important to take precautions to prevent your partner from lifting and falling—activities that could cause trauma to her abdominal area.

What You Can Do:

How cautious should you be? As a general rule:

FIRST TRIMESTER: In the first trimester the uterus is hidden and protected by the abdominal area.

SECOND AND THIRD TRIMESTERS: Once the pregnancy is visually apparent, the slightest fall can cause bleeding in the placenta, a potentially life-threatening condition for both mother and child.

❍ Help your partner avoid lifting any weight in excess of what feels *very light* to *both* of you. What is very light? That will differ from woman to woman. Ideally, lifting the object shouldn't require any effort. Why? Lifting that requires effort may cause further imbalance and a fall. For example, if first trimester wooziness makes her feel uneasy when she walks, the additional front-loaded weight of a heavy grocery bag may cause her to misjudge her steps and fall. By contrast, carrying a grocery bag light enough to carry in one hand may not have this effect.

? What about strangers bumping into her when she uses public transportation? The usual bumping and pushing that occurs on public buses and trains is likely to exert no more pressure than her own hand does when feeling for the baby's movements.

◌ Help your partner with other children. Lifting a small child can be just as strenuous as lifting a heavy bag of groceries, and is just as likely to lead to a tumble. There are also the risks of the child falling on or inadvertently kicking at the abdominal area. For this reason, even if she can lift an older child effortlessly, encourage your partner to hold the child with legs facing away from her abdomen. If the child can stand, ask him or her to climb on a chair to prevent your partner from having to bend.

◌ Think ahead of your partner's missteps. It is very common for women to fall at night, on their way from the bed to the bathroom. Make a point of eyeing the path between these two destinations before bedtime. Clear away objects that she might trip on. Other common falls occur in between meals, when blood sugar is low and dizziness is common. Encourage your partner to snack in between meals to avoid this. Think: *anticipation and prevention.*

? Does any of this mean that you should be afraid to touch your partner's belly and feel the baby's movements? Not at all. Just follow her lead as to what level of touch is comfortable and enjoy the moment.

When to Get More Help:

After the first trimester, report *any fall* or *hard impact* occuring to the pregnancy area. This allows your partner's physician to ask follow-up questions and determine whether it is necessary for your partner to come in for further examination.

The Problem: **Bed Rest Requirements**

The Facts:

Your physician may require your partner to go on partial or complete bed rest for a number of reasons: risk of premature labor, prevention of repeated premature labor; high blood pressure disorder *(hypertension)*, bleeding disorder or slow growth or no growth of the baby.

The most important thing to know about bed rest or partial bed rest is that it is *not voluntary* or self-elected. No woman would choose to submit herself to the extreme boredom and frustration associated with bed rest. Not convinced? Try lying in bed for two days.

The second most important thing about a bed rest order is that it's *not optional.* To achieve the benefits of bed rest (i.e., a healthy, full-term pregnancy), she must actually be *in* bed, in a calm, relaxed mental state. If she is walking around tidying up the house, or if she is in bed, but fretting over the things she *should* be doing, the advantages of bed rest are lost.

What You Can Do:

The best thing you can do when her physician has prescribed bed rest is to make it more likely that she will actually stay in bed and remain relatively relaxed:

☞ Speak with your partner and her physician to ensure that there are no gray areas about what she can or cannot do. Is she on "complete bed rest?" Does she have "bathroom privileges" or "eating privileges?" Can she move around the bedroom? Can she walk around the house? Every point must be clarified with her physician. Your job is to ensure that—despite overwhelming boredom—she sticks to doctor's orders.

○ If she is on "complete bed rest," with no bathroom or kitchen privileges, ensure that there is someone at home caring for her needs, or someone who drops in to ensure that there is food and water within an arm's reach and to help her safely reach the bathroom. If necessary, get her a hand extension device to help her grab out-of-reach items and prevent her from straining.

? What about your older children? Young children can quickly sabotage a well-intentioned bed rest. If you are unavailable, arrange for someone else to care for the child—either at home or off-site.

○ Realize that if there is work to be done, she will get out of bed to do it. Ensure that there is no work to do by soliciting help from family, friends or hired assistance. Alternatively, negotiate with your health-care provider (i.e., insurance or HMO) for coverage of the required help. If you find that none of these options are available to you, talk to her physician about admitting her to the hospital for the duration of her bed rest order.

! It may not surprise you to learn that once her physician admits her into the hospital, your insurance or HMO will be far more willing to cover the expenses associated with proper bed rest at home, including around the clock nursing care, as this is far more economical than a hospital stay.

○ Make her bed more comfortable with soft sheets and a softer mattress. If your existing mattress isn't ideal, consider adding a layer of "egg crate" foam, available at most bed and bath stores.

○ Try to recall any funny movie she enjoyed or intended to see and bring it home on VHS or DVD. Alternatively, if your budget allows, get a few premium cable movie stations for the duration of her bed rest.

- Help her stay connected to the outside world by arranging for her to have a telephone by her bedside. If necessary, bring in a laptop computer and a fax machine—all within arm's reach. If she decides to work while in bed, make sure that her work is light and nonstressful. Ideally, your partner should only work to keep up with the office and avoid boredom, *not* to create stress.

- If she has no office work to keep up with and finds that she cannot bear the boredom of bed rest, consider engaging an *occupational therapist* to help her constructively fill up her many hours in bed.

- If your partner's bed rest is prolonged and her movement is severely restricted, contact your health-care provider (insurance or HMO) and insist that they provide a physical therapist to work with your partner and avoid muscle atrophy. Otherwise she may not be able to stand on her own two feet on the day she goes into labor!

When to Get More Help:

If, despite your best efforts, your partner cannot stay in bed and away from work, as instructed, contact her physician for help. He or she will take time to reemphasize why bed rest is required and the consequences of going against doctor's orders. It may be necessary for your partner to be startled by her physician before she will fully commit to her bed rest orders.

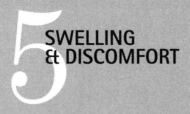

5 SWELLING & DISCOMFORT

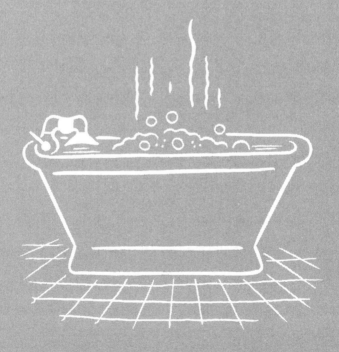

The Problem: **Edema, Water Retention & Swollen Ankles & Hands**

The Facts:

Water retention, or *edema,* is extremely common in late pregnancy because it serves a unique biological function. The retained
water provides a reserve in the likely event that your partner is
unable to eat or drink during labor. Considering that some labor
lasts up to several days and may involve the loss of body fluids,
the reserved water ensures that the baby remains relatively
hydrated.

In today's controlled labor and delivery environment, this
water reserve is not necessary, and merely serves as a nuisance
when the additional water reserve collects in her hands, causing
her fingers to swell to the point where she cannot remove
her ring(s), and in her ankles, making it uncomfortable for her
to walk.

Why does edema collect in the hands and ankles? Actually,
edema collects in soft tissue throughout the body, but especially
at the lowest point of your partner's extremities—her hands
and ankles.

? How can you tell if she is retaining water? Push your
index finger against the bone of her ankle. If your finger
creates an indentation that takes a few seconds to fade,
then she has edema. This test is also a good way to
monitor her edema.

What You Can Do:

Help for swollen hands and feet breaks down into bringing down
the swelling and taking precautions to make her more comfortable in her swollen state.

BRINGING DOWN HER SWELLING:

◯ Encourage her to supplement her diet with *magnesium glyci-nate, magnesium gluconate, magnesium citrate, magnesium aspartate* or another fast-absorbing magnesium available from your local health food store. Suggest that she take the recom-mended dosage with food and slowly increase her intake every few days until her swelling decreases. Reduce her dosage if she experiences fatigue, muscle weakness or diarrhea.

◯ If your partner is taking magnesium, consider adding a good vitamin B complex to her supplement program. A dosage of 25 to 50 milligrams, taken once daily will increase the effi-ciency of her magnesium supplement and also serve as an energy booster. Also try 100 milligrams of vitamin B_6, taken twice daily.

◯ *Evening primrose oil* capsules, also available in your health food store, can help bring down your partner's swelling. The active ingredient, *gamma linolenic acid,* is the helpful com-ponent of these capsules. A dose containing 125 milligrams of gamma linolenic acid should be taken with breakfast.

◯ Make your partner a morning smoothie that includes parsley, dandelion leaf, cilantro, dill, cucumber or watermelon. All of these are natural diuretics and are helpful in reducing swelling. Add these ingredients to the basic *Quick Protein Smoothie* recipe in the appendix of this guidebook (page 199).

◯ Encourage your partner to lie down on her side. The horizontal position promotes the reabsorption of the retained water.

◯ Draw a *warm,* but not a hot, bath for your partner. Bath water should not exceed 98 degrees Fahrenheit. Exposure to bath water heated above 98 degrees Fahrenheit may increase the rate of birth defects and, in advanced pregnancy, may lead to premature contractions and delivery. Help her climb in and

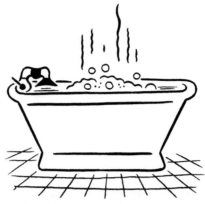

immerse her body and legs in water—all the way up to her neck. Keep her company or stay close by, as she is likely to require a bathroom trip every 15 to 20 minutes, and will need your help for a safe exit and reimmersion. The bath will help move water from unwanted areas—like her hands and feet—to areas beneficial to the baby, including the amniotic fluid.

○ Unless otherwise indicated by her physician, it is not necessary to restrict salt consumption simply because your partner is retaining water. Sodium should only be restricted when it is obvious that water retention increases immediately after she has eaten salty food.

MAKING HER MORE COMFORTABLE:

○ Encourage her to wear loose-fitting clothing.

○ Suggest that she purchase new shoes. Although your partner may prefer thongs and slip-ons that don't inhibit the width of her feet, athletic shoes that provide ankle support are best. Purchase a size that fits her regardless of whether she will be able to wear them after her pregnancy.

○ You will find that your partner's level of edema rises and falls very quickly. The shoes she wore yesterday may not fit her today. However unbelievable, give her the benefit of the doubt—she's not imagining her condition.

- If your partner is prone to swelling in her hands, encourage her to remove her rings until after her delivery. Her edema will become more dramatic as her delivery date draws closer, to the point where she may not be able to remove her rings at all. It is not uncommon for women to have to cut off their rings in order to alleviate the pressure of edema.

When to Get More Help:

If your partner develops edema in the first half of her pregnancy, notify her physician.

If, during the second half of her pregnancy, your partner's onset of edema includes headache, blurry vision or pain on the right side, below her rib cage, immediately report this to her physician.

The Problem: **Carpal Tunnel Syndrome**

The Facts:

Believe it or not, carpal tunnel syndrome in pregnancy is directly related to water retention. How? One of the nerves that controls hand function is enveloped by a circular ligament at the wrist. When a pregnant woman's body—including this ligament— retains water, the swollen ligament puts pressure on this key hand-controlling nerve and creates pain, pressure and decreased mobility in the fingers.

What You Can Do:

Helping your partner avoid water retention (which will also diminish swollen hands and ankles) will assist in reducing her carpal tunnel syndrome discomfort:

- If your partner is prone to swelling in her hands, encourage her to supplement her diet with *magnesium glycinate, magnesium gluconate, magnesium citrate, magnesium aspartate* or another fast-absorbing magnesium available from your local health food store. Suggest that she take begin taking the suggested dosage with food and slowly increase her intake every few days until her swelling and pain decrease. Reduce her dosage if she experiences fatigue, muscle weakness or diarrhea.

- If your partner is taking magnesium, consider adding a good vitamin B complex to her supplement program. A dosage of 25 to 50 milligrams, taken once daily will increase the efficiency of her magnesium supplement and also serve as an energy booster. Also try 100 milligrams of vitamin B_6, taken twice daily.

- *Evening primrose oil* capsules, the key ingredient of which is *gamma linolenic acid*, are also available in your health food store and can help bring down your partner's wrist swelling and discomfort. Suggest she take 125 milligrams with breakfast.

- Make your partner a morning smoothie that includes parsley, dandelion leaf, cilantro, dill, cucumber or watermelon. All of these are natural diuretics, and are therefore helpful in reducing her wrist swelling. Consider adding these ingredients to the *Easy Vegetable Soup* recipe in the appendix of this guidebook (page 200).

- Encourage your partner to lie down on her side. The horizontal position promotes the reabsorption of the retained water.

- Draw a *warm,* but not a hot, bath for your partner. Bath water should not exceed 98 degrees Fahrenheit. Exposure to bath water heated above 98 degrees Fahrenheit may increase the rate of birth defects and, in advanced pregnancy, may lead to premature contractions and delivery. Help her climb in and immerse her body and legs in water—all the way up to her neck. Keep her company or stay close by, as she is likely to require a bathroom trip every 15 to 20 minutes, and will need your help for a safe exit and reimmersion. This bath will help move water from her wrists to areas beneficial to the baby, including the amniotic fluid.

- Unless otherwise indicated by her physician, it is not necessary to restrict salt consumption simply because your partner is retaining water. Sodium should only be restricted when it is obvious that wrist swelling and pain increases immediately after she has eaten salty food.

- Many women who have been advised to avoid medication in pregnancy find that acupuncture can be helpful in alleviating painful carpel tunnel syndrome symptoms.

- Bracing the wrist can also be helpful. A pharmacist or orthopedic surgeon can provide your partner with a removable wrist brace.

When to Get More Help:

Consult your partner's physician for a referral when your partner's wrist pain is so great that she cannot perform her daily tasks.

The Problem: **Hemorrhoids & Varicose Veins**

The Facts:

Hemorrhoids are an aggravation of the rectal veins. They occur in pregnancy due to:

- constipation,

- pressure by the uterus,

- stagnation of blood caused by decreased activity, and

- the presence of the hormone *progesterone,* which relaxes the vein muscles.

Many of these factors are also the cause of varicose veins, a condition in which the aggravated veins are visible on the pregnant women's legs.

While varicose veins will be easy to detect, your partner may be uncomfortable about admitting that she is suffering from hemorrhoids. Generally, if she is suffering from constipation and varicose veins, she is also likely to have hemorrhoids.

What You Can Do:

AVOIDING VARICOSE VEINS AND HEMORRHOIDS:

- By helping to prevent her episodes of constipation, you will also help her significantly reduce the development of hemorrhoids and varicose veins. For more information, see the *Constipation* section of this guidebook (page 103).

- Encourage her to avoid the development of hemorrhoids and varicose veins by staying active. Invite her on a slow, romantic evening walk or encourage her to swim.

- Encourage her to avoid lifting items that cause her to strain. Help her by coming along or doing the grocery shopping, a common opportunity for women to ignore heavy lifting restrictions. If you have another child, consider whether he or she is too heavy for your partner's condition. For more information on these restrictions, see the *Heavy Lifting & Falling during Pregnancy* section of this guidebook (page 87).

TREATING VARICOSE VEINS AND HEMORRHOIDS:

○ To reduce varicose veins, see your pharmacist for a pair of special pregnancy support hose or leggings. Encourage your partner to put them on in the morning and remove them at night. She may sleep in them during the day if she is on bed rest. If she feels that these support hose are too tight, visit your pharmacist for another size and pressure strength.

○ Visit your health food store for a variety of natural varicose vein remedies, including *nettles* and *oatstraw* teas and a homeopathic remedy called *Hamamelis 30X,* to be used as directed.

○ Visit your local pharmacy for creams containing zinc, such as zinc oxide, to be applied topically to the affected area.

○ For hemorrhoids during pregnancy, try to avoid the common over-the-counter medications. Look for natural alternatives. For example, see your pharmacist for witch hazel "tucks" that will adhere to your partner's affected area.

When to Get More Help:

If her hemorrhoids become painful, notify her physician. If they become extremely painful, ask her physician for a referral to a colon-rectal specialist or gastroenterologist.

If her varicose veins become red, hot, and painful and you can see a red line on the back of her legs, from her ankles to her calves or thighs, notify her physician immediately.

The Problem: **Constipation**

The Facts:

Constipation in pregnancy is caused by:

> ▶ a relaxing of the muscular activity of the bowels by the hormone *progesterone*,
>
> ▶ the pressure of the baby on the bowels,
>
> ▶ the body's relative decrease in thyroid function,
>
> ▶ dehydration, and
>
> ▶ lack of sufficient fiber in your partner's diet.

Consistent constipation will make your partner's pregnancy experience more uncomfortable. She will be also more likely to develop hemorrhoids, only adding to her discomfort. The more you do to decrease and prevent her constipation, the more pleasant her pregnancy will be.

What You Can Do:

LIGHT CONSTIPATION AND CONSTIPATION PREVENTION:

◌ Your partner may be suffering from constipation, but may feel uncomfortable about mentioning it. Asking her whether she is "having trouble going to the bathroom" is a polite way to determine whether she is suffering from this problem.

◌ Encourage her to drink at least 8 to 12 glasses of water per day.

◌ Encourage her to consume fruits, vegetables and other fiber-rich foods.

◌ Invite your partner for slow daily walks. Activity reduces constipation.

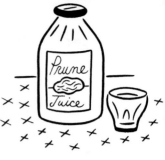

- Pick up prunes and prune juice at your local market. Encourage her to drink or eat this great natural remedy with her breakfast. Alternatively, add either to the *Quick Protein Smoothie* recipe in the appendix of this guidebook (page 199).

- *Magnesium* is nature's constipation buster. Visit your local health food store for *magnesium carbonate, magnesium oxide* or another form of magnesium that is easily absorbed by the body. Encourage her to supplement her diet with 250 milligrams, twice daily, slowly increasing her dosage every few days until her stool becomes soft. The more pregnant your partner is, the more magnesium she is likely to need.

- Ask your partner to speak to her physician about her thyroid level. If her thyroid function is low or on the low side of "normal," optimizing her level will alleviate constipation. Ask her physician to check her *Free T3* and *Free T4* levels, rather than simply doing a standard thyroid test, for more accurate results in pregnancy.

IF YOUR PARTNER HAS NOT HAD A BOWEL MOVEMENT FOR TWO TO THREE DAYS:

- Visit your local health food store for a bottle of food-quality mineral oil, a natural stool softener. Encourage your partner to drink 30 cc units or one or two teaspoons once daily, for no longer than two consecutive days.

- Additionally, your pharmacist can provide you with *glycerin* suppositories to be used three times daily.

- Finally, your partner may also use an over-the-counter enema, available from your pharmacist.

When to Get More Help:

If your partner has not had a bowel movement in three days, despite the suggestions provided above, or if the constipation is associated with abdominal cramps, contact her physician.

6 PREGNANCY RESTRICTIONS

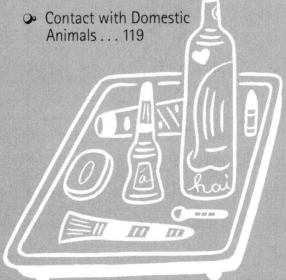

The Problem: **Restrictions on Sex**

The Facts:

There is no medical reason to avoid sex during pregnancy. With a few slight variations, your sex lives can proceed as before. However, you will find that your partner is softer, more lubricated and less tight.

What You Can Do:

Consider the following as general guidelines:

FIRST TRIMESTER: Unless otherwise instructed by her physician, there are no restrictions on sexual contact during the first three months of pregnancy.

SECOND TRIMESTER: Avoid positions in which she is on her abdomen or on her back. Lying on her abdomen puts pressure on the pregnancy, while lying on her back decreases the blood flow to the baby by up to 30 percent. Instead, approach from the side or from the back. Deep penetration will not hurt the baby or put the pregnancy in jeopardy.

THIRD TRIMESTER: Follow the same position guidelines as in the second trimester. While sex at the very end of the ninth month *may* cause your partner's water to break "prematurely," this is not a problem. Why? Since your child is fully mature, your partner will simply proceed with a normal labor and delivery.

? Some men feel that their organ is making contact with the baby during sex—especially in the third trimester. Is this true? Generally not. While *possible* at the end of the ninth month, *if* your partner's cervix is dilated and effaced, this type of contact won't affect the baby either way.

You may find that she feels tired, self-conscious about her new shape or that the discomforts of early and late pregnancy make her disinterested in sex. Some women avoid sex because they feel protective of the baby. A change in sexual relations during pregnancy should not be seen as a shaking of the foundations of your relationship. Work around the various roadblocks as follows:

- Take over a few of your partner's morning chores to give her an additional hour or two of sleep.

- Reassure her that sex cannot harm the baby. Encourage her to speak to her physician about this, or provide her with reading materials on the subject.

- Reestablish intimacy by lying close to her and touching her stomach. Put your ear against her stomach to listen to the baby.

- Offer to massage her feet with a massage lotion. Once her feet are done, reapply the massage lotion to your hands and work your way up, massaging her legs until you reach her torso. This massage can be relaxing and inspiring to your partner.

- If you find that your partner has no interest in intercourse, be understanding. Then pick a day when she is less tired, offer a massage, and then ask her to return the favor.

? Some men find that *they* lose interest in sex during pregnancy, despite their partner's interest. Many men are concerned about hurting the baby or find themselves less attracted to a new version of their partner's physique. Consider taking a step back. Recognize that sex will not hurt the baby, but that a lack of physical attention at a time when she is feeling self-conscious may hurt your partner. Consider a few of the suggestions described above for finding ways to connect with your partner on an intimate level.

⚬ Recognize that whatever attraction has waned during her pregnancy will no doubt return once she is no longer complaining of aches and pains.

When to Get More Help:

If your partner experiences pain during intercourse, or bleeding or cramping after intercourse, it's time to call her physician. He or she will tell you whether it is necessary to call the next time similar bleeding occurs.

Other symptoms requiring a doctor's attention include foul-smelling discharge (a sign of bacterial infection), a foul smell on the penis (another sign of bacterial infection), or if your partner's water breaks during or after intercourse.

The Problem: **Exposure to High Temperatures**

(Also see the *Cold & Flu* section of this guidebook [page 122].)

The Facts:

Exposing the pregnant body to heat, including fevers, hot showers, hot tubs, saunas, stuffy rooms, hot exercise rooms, overexercise without proper hydration and beauty treatments that involve heat is harmful to the well-being of the pregnancy. Heat may increase the rate of birth defects and, in advanced pregnancy, may lead to premature contractions and delivery.

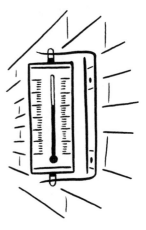

What You Can Do:

◌ Whenever your partner exercises and her skin feels hot to either of you, encourage her to recognize that her body is becoming overheated. Suggest that she lower her activity level and drink additional fluids as she exercises.

◌ Prepare her a natural sports drink by simply adding honey and sea salt to the water she drinks.

◌ Ensure that she avoids baths, hot tubs, and showers with temperatures above 98 degrees Fahrenheit.

◌ Ensure that she avoids saunas, body wraps and any other beauty treatments that generate heat.

◌ Ensure that she avoids exercise classes conducted in heated or stuffy rooms, including stationary bicycle and heated yoga classes.

◐ If your partner develops a fever, bring down her temperature with cold drinks and a shower, and see the *Cold & Flu* section of this guidebook (page 122) for more specific information.

When to Get More Help:

Any time she develops a fever over 100 degrees that does not respond to the cooling measures, contact her physician.

The Problem: **Skin Disorders in Pregnancy**

The Facts:

In general, your partner's skin will be more sensitive during pregnancy, and her skin may actually change during this time. Some sensitivities and changes are normal; others are not.

Normal skin changes include an increase in oiliness, a patchy discoloration of the face, the appearance of a dark line between the pubic bone and the navel and spiderlike bursts of vessels, sometimes called "spider veins." Most of these conditions will fade after the pregnancy.

It is also normal for her skin to become more sensitive to soaps, beauty products and household cleaning agents used prior to pregnancy. For more information, see the *Safety of Beauty Products* section of this guidebook (page 115).

What You Can Do:

◌ If your partner takes medication for any skin condition—by mouth or external application—advise her to discontinue her use until after she has consulted with her physician and the doctor who prescribed the medication.

◌ If she uses over-the-counter skin medication, suggest that she bring these products with her the next time she sees her physician and, unless absolutely essential, discontinue use until the medication has been approved.

◌ Encourage her to help reduce her skin irritation by drinking 8 to 12 glasses of water per day.

◌ If she experiences irritation, suggest that she discontinue using soaps with artificial color and fragrance. Bring home a beautifully wrapped bar of unscented, uncolored glycerin soap—the most pure form of soap. Encourage her to wash her face, body and undergarments with this soap.

- Many personal care products have packaging that indicates that they are "pure" or "natural." If she develops an irritation while using these products, suggest that she discontinue use regardless of the assurances on the packaging.

- Encourage her to stock up on moisturizers and other personal care products that are designed for sensitive skin, and those products that have fewer unnecessary additives.

When to Get More Help:

If she experiences sudden skin changes, such as reddening or itching, that spread to more than a small portion of her skin, contact her physician or a dermatologist for a consultation.

Gradual skin changes that are not painful should be addressed during routine pregnancy appointments.

The Problem: The Safety of Beauty Products

The Facts:

While beauty products alone—soaps, creams and treatments—are not problematic during pregnancy, many beauty products are laden with chemicals that can cause problems.

A woman's skin becomes much more sensitive in pregnancy and more likely to develop allergic reactions to products that caused no problems prior to pregnancy. Beyond this, because skin is so absorbent, the chemical makeup of all products used—even those used on hair and skin—ultimately transfers to the baby.

What You Can Do:

- Allow your partner to decide what she is comfortable using on her body. Due to the body changes associated with pregnancy, she may need her tried-and-true beauty products to make her feel attractive.

- If she does develop an irritation, suggest that she stop using any product that she relates with the irritation, even if the label describes it as "pure."

- Encourage her to use soaps, shampoos and other beauty products that are made without artificial color or fragrance. Look for natural substitutes at your local health food store.

- Bring home a beautifully wrapped package of glycerin soap produced without artificial color or fragrance. This type of soap

is the least likely to produce an allergic reaction and is ideal for washing her skin and undergarments.

○» Discourage her from becoming too concerned about what will or will not harm the baby. Suggest that she do the best that she can. After all, with the amount of pollutants and other chemicals modern living exposes us to daily, a little perfumed soap is unlikely to make much of a difference. Suggest that her safest course is to keep things simple and avoid those products she can live without.

When to Get More Help:

If she has used a beauty product and developed an allergic reaction, discontinue use and, if the irritation continues, bring it to the attention of her physician.

The Problem: The Safety of Beauty Treatments

The Facts:

As with beauty products, and with a few exceptions, beauty treatments are only objectionable to the extent they cause irritation and expose your partner's body—and the baby—to unnecessary chemical substances.

What You Can Do:

- Since the physical changes associated with pregnancy very often cause women to feel less attractive, encourage her to continue pampering herself with beauty treatments that do not expose her to high temperatures or harmful chemicals.

- When possible, suggest a "natural" alternative, such as natural hair color or nail "buffing" for fingernails.

- Which beauty treatments are safe?

  - Body waxing, including bikini waxing

  - Facial and hair bleaching, so long as she avoids bleach fumes by wearing a mask

  - Hair styling, so long as she avoids hair spray fumes

  - Hair color, but vegetable dyes or hennas are preferable

  - Manicures and pedicures, but suggest that she avoid acrylic nails and bring her own nail file, cuticle trimmer, pumice stone or callous shaver

  - Facials, but suggest a natural product facial or those designed for "sensitive skin"

  - Massages

! Encourage her to avoid body wraps, mud baths, saunas and hot tubs, as the increased body temperature associated with these treatments is harmful in pregnancy.

◦ On the other hand, massages are a wonderful way for pregnant women to relax, increase the lymphatic blood flow, ease back pain, leg cramps and aching feet. Surprise her with a home massage (by you or a professional massage therapist) or a visit to a local day spa. Pregnant women in their second and third trimesters should not lie on their backs or stomachs during massage. Many massage therapists use specially designed pillows that allow pregnant women to lie on their stomachs without putting pressure on the baby. Otherwise she should lie on her side.

When to Get More Help:

Absent heat treatments, the likelihood of harming a baby with beauty treatments is low. Nonetheless, when in doubt, encourage her to postpone the treatment and seek the advice of her physician.

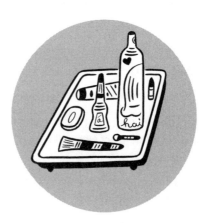

The Problem: Contact with Domestic Animals

The Facts:

Contact with household pets requires added attention when your partner is pregnant. In some cases her contact will be severely restricted, while other instances simply require added attention to avoid a fall or other injury.

What You Can Do:

- **Cats.** The feces of household cats may contain a bacteria called *toxoplasmosis*, which is harmful to the developing baby. If you do not already do so, take over the duty of cleaning out the cat's litter box and suggest that your partner limit her contact with this pet. If you have a cat, ask her physician to test your partner for toxoplasmosis antibodies prior to or at the beginning of pregnancy.

- **Dogs.** The second and third trimesters of pregnancy require pregnant women to be especially careful about slips and falls. Often walking a large dog—especially when other dogs or animals are nearby—may cause a fall. Discourage her from walking large dogs alone and engaging in rough play. Similarly, carrying or holding small dogs may conflict with restrictions on lifting objects in pregnancy. It is also possible for a small dog to kick at the pregnancy area when he would like to be let go. Discourage her from carrying or holding a dog on her lap. For more information, see the *Heavy Lifting & Falling during Pregnancy* section of this guidebook (page 87). Always ensure that she avoids animal feces.

☙ **Flea shampoos.** Many flea shampoos and related products contain toxins that will be absorbed by your partner's skin as she bathes or pets the treated animal. This exposure is increased if your pet sleeps with you on the bed. If possible, refrain from treating your pet with flea shampoos and dips for the duration of the pregnancy.

When to Get More Help:

Consult her physician with specific pet-related concerns.

If she develops a rash that she attributes to her contact with pets, contact her physician.

7
ILLNESS & INFECTION

The Problem: Cold & Flu

The Facts:

While colds and flus are common in pregnancy, your treatment of these ailments will not be. Pregnant women cannot rely on the same over-the-counter cold and flu medications as non-pregnant women. Moreover, if your partner runs a fever, treatment of the fever will take precedence over the treatment of any other symptom.

? **Why treat fevers first? Studies indicate that the babies of women who experienced fever in the first trimester of pregnancy suffer from an increased risk of congenital heart defects.**

What You Can Do:

IF SHE HAS A FEVER:

❧ Keep her temperature under 100.4 degrees Fahrenheit by giving her cold beverages and placing her in a cold bath or shower. While she is in the bath, keep her company or stay close by, as she will need your help to safely exit.

❧ While using *acetaminophen* (commonly known as Tylenol) to bring down your partner's fever has been known to be harmful to the liver, simply adding a supplement called NAC *(N-Acetyl-L-Cysteine)* to your *acetaminophen* dosage will remedy this problem. To bring down her fever safely, give your partner one or two regular strength *acetaminophen* pills every four to six hours, and take one 250 milligram NAC pill for every *acetaminophen* pill taken.

❧ Encourage your partner to take time out of her schedule to rest, even if she wouldn't take the time to do so in her non-pregnant state.

- Visit your local health food store for natural cold remedies, including:

  - vitamin C, 10 grams per day for no more than one week,

  - elderberry extract,

  - colostrum extract,

  - garlic pills,

  - zinc lozenges or spray, and

  - echinacea *without* goldenseal.

! **Do not give your partner a natural supplement called *goldenseal*, often packaged with *echinacea*, as this herb has been known to cause contractions.**

- Encourage your partner to drink at least 8 to 12 glasses of water per day.

IF SHE HAS A COLD OR FLU WITH NO FEVER:

- Follow the last three suggestions above.

When to Get More Help:

Contact your partner's physician when you detect her fever. Call again if your partner's fever does not respond to treatment, rises higher or affects her breathing.

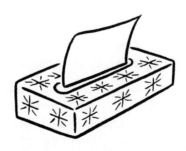

The Problem: Acid Reflux, Acidic Stomach & Indigestion

The Facts:

One of the miseries of pregnancy—particularly late pregnancy—is acid reflux, a condition sometimes described as an acidic or sour stomach.

Why does this happen? As the baby and uterus grow, they squeeze the gastrointestinal track so that acid from the stomach is pushed toward the esophagus. Moreover, the presence of the pregnancy hormone *progesterone* causes the *esophageal sphincter,* the organ charged with blocking acid from rising back up the esophagus, to relax to the point of being less effective. This causes the same painful acid reflux condition that many men suffer from.

What You Can Do:

○ Encourage her to eat relatively small meals more frequently.

○ Ideally, your partner should stay away from foods that exacerbate her acid reflux. While the offending foods will be different for each woman, it is generally helpful for her to avoid foods that are heavy or served in large portions.

○ Discourage her from lying down after she eats. Invite her to take a short walk with you. If she must rest after a meal, be sure that her torso is propped up vertically to stop acid from rising up in her esophagus.

○ When she does sleep, help her prop up her head with pillows, so that her torso is elevated above her stomach.

○ Although over-the-counter antacids may help control the discomfort of acid reflux, they tend to neutralize *all* acid in the gastrointestinal tract—including the acid that the stomach uses to digest food. Without sufficient stomach acid, food tends to rot, and indigestion develops. Before turning to more common antacids, look for natural alternatives (i.e., homeopathic and herbal remedies), including *fennel seed tea,* at your local health food store.

When to Get More Help:

If your partner is not able to control her acid reflux and it becomes intolerable, consult her physician for assistance. In those extreme situations when prescription antacids are recommended, encourage your partner to use them sparingly, and only at night.

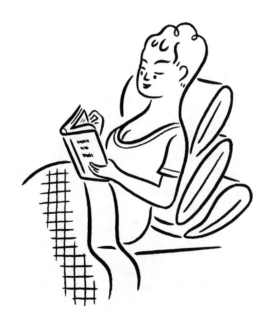

The Problem: **Stomachache, Belching or Gas**

The Facts:

During pregnancy, the gastrointestinal track is more sensitive, because it serves as the protective barrier between the outside world and the baby. For this reason, pregnant women may experience more frequent stomachaches, belching or gas—despite the fact that they are eating better food and more of it!

What You Can Do:

- Make note of her digestive complaints and their frequency. Encourage her to do the same.

- If she becomes bloated immediately after she eats, she may lack *hydrochloric acid.* This oral supplement can be found at your local health food store under the name *betaine.* Encourage her to take one or two standard dosage pills at the beginning of each meal. You will know that her dosage is too high if she gets heartburn.

- Consistent gas or bloating can also be a symptom of a lack of digestive enzymes. Visit your local health food store for a digestive enzyme supplement to be taken at the end of her meals. Additionally, taking "friendly" bacteria, such as *lacto-bacillus acidophilus* supplements, with her meal may help prevent future indigestion and bloating. Use as directed.

- On the flip side, bloating and gas may also result from an over-growth of "bad" yeast or bacteria in the gastrointestinal track. This condition is made worse by the high level of progesterone found in your partner's pregnant body. An easy treatment for this is pure oregano oil, found at your local health food store.

Suggest that your partner drink four drops in a quarter glass of water or juice, three times daily.

When to Get More Help:

If your partner experiences severe pain, constant diarrhea or vomiting, contact her doctor.

The Problem: **Diarrhea & Food Poisoning**

The Facts:

Pregnant women often experience more frequent bouts of diarrhea and food poisoning, in part because their bodies are more sensitive to improperly stored foods and chemical food additives. At the slightest sign of danger, the pregnant body expels food in an attempt to rid itself of abnormal bacteria and viral infections. While diarrhea and other symptoms of food poisoning are not problematic, the resulting dehydration, electrolyte imbalance and malnutrition may lead to fatigue, diminished nutrition for the baby and even the onset of premature contractions.

What You Can Do:

◦ Help her avoid dehydration by encouraging her to drink as much water as she will tolerate. Pregnant women should drink 8 to 12 glasses of water daily.

◦ Help her restore her electrolyte balance by providing her with natural versions of sports drinks, made without artificial coloring and available at your local health food store. Alternatively, make your own natural sports drink by adding sea salt and honey to water.

◦ If you find that she is not able to keep down the water she drinks, feed her ice cubes or smaller amounts of water—even if it's only one teaspoon at a time.

When to Get More Help:

Contact her physician if the diarrhea or vomiting does not improve within 24 hours.

The Problem: Frequent Urination

(Also see the *Urinary Tract & Bladder Infections* [page 131],
Kidney Infection [page 134] and *Vaginal Infection* [page 136]
sections of this guidebook.)

The Facts:

Frequent urination, particularly at night, is caused by the enlarged
uterus pressing against your partner's bladder. It is also one of
the ways your partner's body trains her to sleep very lightly, so
that later she will be able to hear the baby crying and awake to
feed every two hours in the baby's first few weeks of life.

What You Can Do:

◌ There is very little you can do about your partner's natural
tendency to urinate more frequently during the night. If she is
frustrated by this condition,
remind her that this is a natural
process that serves a biological
purpose. Discourage her from
cutting down her fluid intake
in an attempt to curb nightly
bathroom trips, as this could
adversely affect her pregnancy.
Pregnant women should drink
8 to 12 glasses of water per day.

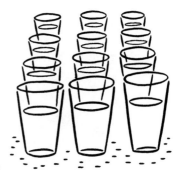

◌ So long as bladder infections have been ruled out by her
physician, discourage your partner from becoming concerned
about her frequent urination.

◌ To decrease the chances that your partner's nightly bathroom
trips will prevent her from sleeping through the night, see
the suggestions in the *Insomnia* section of this guidebook
(page 51).

When to Get More Help:

Encourage your partner to schedule an appointment for a urine culture any time she experiences:

- more frequent urination than usual,

- pain during urination, or

- a feeling that she cannot fully empty her bladder when urinating.

The Problem: Urinary Tract & Bladder Infections

(Also see the *Frequent Urination* [page 129] and *Kidney Infection* [page 134] sections in this guidebook.)

The Facts:

Another reason for frequent urination in pregnancy is the development of bladder and urinary tract infections, some of which may not show all of their symptoms, but all of which can lead to an increased risk of premature delivery and kidney infection. Bladder and urinary tract infections are more common during pregnancy because:

▶ the hormones associated with pregnancy dilate the bladder and tube that connects the bladder and the kidneys (the *ureter*), causing urine to collect in the bladder and increase the occurrence of infection, and

▶ the increased lubrication of the vagina and clumsiness associated with your partner's growing size make it more difficult to maintain hygiene, which increases the likelihood of infection.

! **Another form of bladder infection typical to pregnancy can develop without any of the symptoms described above** *(asymptomatic bacteriuria).* **This infection is often related to premature labor. For this reason, many physicians' offices do routine tests for this condition in the second trimester.**

What You Can Do:

◦ Encourage your partner to schedule an appointment for a urine culture any time she experiences:

▶ more frequent urination than usual,

▶ pain during urination, or

▶ a feeling that she cannot fully empty her bladder when urinating.

! In pregnancy, more than ever, your partner should insist on coming into the doctor's office for a culture, rather than having her physician prescribe an antibiotic over the phone. The right antibiotic must be matched with the right bacteria.

☞ Many times a vaginal infection is the source of your partner's bladder infection. For this reason, always encourage your partner to request a vaginal culture with her urine culture.

☞ To lessen the chance of her developing a bladder or kidney infection, encourage her to drink between 8 to 12 glasses of water per day. Drinking lots of fluid can be a preventive miracle.

☞ Encourage her to supplement her diet with "friendly" bacteria, such as *Lactobacillus acidophilus,* available at your local health food store. This common nutritional supplement will arm her gastrointestinal tract with normal flora and hinder the development of bladder, kidney and urinary tract infections.

☞ Ensure that your partner receives a routine bladder culture in the second trimester to rule out asymptomatic bladder infections.

☞ Consider visiting your local health food store for fresh cranberries, unsweetened cranberry juice or *nettles tea,* all helpful for the prevention and treatment of bladder and urinary tract infections.

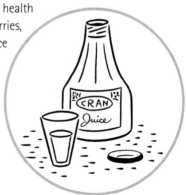

When to Get More Help:

Painful urination should always be brought to the attention of a physician.

If your partner has seen her physician and the treatment prescribed does not improve her condition within 72 hours, contact her physician again.

The Problem: **Kidney Infection**

(Also see the *Frequent Urination* [page 129] and *Urinary Tract & Bladder Infections* [page 131] sections of this guidebook.)

The Facts:

Because bladder infections in pregnancy may not show obvious symptoms, it is common for these infections to have spread to the kidneys by the time your partner is diagnosed. This is a serious concern, in light of the fact that the late treatment of kidney infections could contribute to a permanent loss of partial kidney function.

What You Can Do:

○ Encourage your partner to request an examination to rule out kidney infection any time she experiences:

▶ fever, and

▶ back pain just above the kidneys, at the bottom of her rib cage.

○ Encourage your partner to request an examination to rule out kidney infection any time treatment for a bladder infection does not clear up symptoms within 72 hours.

○ To lessen the chance of her developing a kidney infection, encourage her to drink water. Ideally, your partner should consume 8 to 12 glasses of water per day. Drinking plenty of fluid is a must and can be a preventive miracle.

○ Encourage her to supplement her diet with "friendly" bacteria, such as *Lactobacillus acidophilus,* available at your local health food store. This common nutritional supplement will arm her gastrointestinal tract with normal flora and hinder the development of bladder, kidney and urinary tract infections.

When to Get More Help:

Painful urination should always be brought to the attention of a physician.

In those situations where your partner experiences fever, back pain or shortness of breath, *with or without urinary pain,* do not hesitate to call her physician or to visit the emergency room. Extremely rarely, kidney infection may be associated with a breathing disorder that demands medical attention.

The Problem: **Vaginal Infection**

(Also see the *Urinary Tract & Bladder Infections* [page 131] and *Kidney Infection* [page 134] sections of this guidebook.)

The Facts:

Women are prone to vaginal infections regardless of pregnancy. Women are *more* likely to develop vaginal infection in pregnancy due to:

▶ increased yeast infections due to an increase in the hormone *progesterone,* and

▶ increased bacterial infections due to a higher level of vaginal lubrication and size-related clumsiness, which makes it difficult for your partner to maintain proper hygiene in pregnancy.

Pregnant women also experience an increased allergic sensitivity to chemicalized soaps, perfumes and detergents, which may result in itching and other symptoms similar to those of vaginal infection.

? Are vaginal infections problematic during pregnancy? Yes and no. Yeast infection and allergic reaction don't affect the well-being of the pregnancy—they are simply annoying and can be easily and safely treated by your partner's physician. However, a bacterial infection in the vagina can cause problems with the pregnancy. For example:

▶ Common infections such as *bacterial vaginosis* and *Gardinella* may cause premature labor, early breakage of the water and infection after the birth. While non-pregnant women with these conditions are often treated with vaginal suppositories or cream, pregnancy requires the use of oral medication for more aggressive treatment.

▶ Another infection, called *mycoplasma,* is characterized by yellow vaginal discharge and may lead to miscarriage,

premature delivery, premature water breakage and infection after the delivery.

▶ A *chlamydia* infection can cause permanent infant
blindness during delivery.

▶ Finally, *vaginal beta strep,* the vaginal version of the
bacteria that causes strep throat, could lead to a fatal
infection in some infants. Women with a beta strep infection require an antibiotic treatment four hours prior to
vaginal delivery to prevent the spread of the infection to
the baby.

What You Can Do:

◑ It is common for women to have an increase in vaginal discharge during pregnancy. Healthy discharge is white, liquidy,
acidic but not foul smelling. If you notice yellowish, foul-
smelling or white flaky discharge, encourage your partner to
call her physician's office for an appointment.

◑ Most harmful bacterial infections grow when the vagina has
lost its own protective bacteria. For this reason, when your
partner goes in for a vaginal culture, encourage her to ask her
physician to measure her *normal* bacteria, as well. If her
normal bacteria levels are low, visit your local health food store
for *Lactobacillus acidophilus* suppositories, made especially for
the vagina. Use as directed.

◑ Obtaining results for your partner's vaginal culture should only
take three days. If your partner has a culture taken and does
not receive a call within three days, contact her physician's
office for the results.

◑ If your partner has yellow discharge or other symptoms of
bacterial infection but her test came out negative, insist that
she return to her physician for a second culture that specifically tests for the infections listed above. It is common for
general cultures to miss more specific infections.

- Four weeks before your partner is due to deliver, a copy of her medical chart will be transferred to the labor and delivery ward of the hospital. Nevertheless, if you know that your partner has the *beta strep* bacteria, remind her physician *and* the hospital staff of this condition—*just in case.* Make sure that she receives the appropriate antibiotic treatment (usually by IV) at least four hours prior to her delivery.

- To help your partner prevent yeast infection, encourage her to cut down on sweets, processed carbohydrates (i.e., breads, pastas, etc.), vinegar and aged cheese.

- Alternatively, help further prevent yeast infections by visiting your local health food store for a small vile of oregano oil or grapefruit extract. Drinking 4 drops of oregano oil in four ounces of juice or water, or 15 drops of grapefruit extract in eight ounces of water or juice, three times daily, can significantly reduce the development of yeast infection. If the flavor of juice does not adequately mask the strong scent and flavor of these oils, try replacing juice with applesauce.

- Loose-fitting clothing that allows for air circulation can also reduce the development of yeast infection.

- To prevent the allergic reactions that cause itching and other symptoms associated with vaginal infections, bring home a bar of the purest, uncolored, unscented glycerin soap you can find. Although it may seem like a strange gift, washing her body and her undergarments with this soap will decrease allergic reactions.

- To help alleviate the significant itching associated with yeast infection or allergic reaction, apply vitamin E oil, honey, *colostrum cream,* prepared oatmeal or the oil removed from capsules of *evening primrose oil* to the area where your partner itches most, usually the vulva. All of these are available at your local health food store. As a last resort, 1 percent *hydro-*

cortisone cream, available over-the-counter, can also be helpful in reducing itching.

When to Get More Help:

In the case of vaginal infections, it is extremely unusual to require immediate, late-night help from her physician or the hospital emergency room. If you suspect that your partner has a vaginal infection, wait until the following morning to arrange for an appointment.

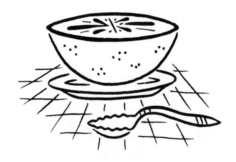

The Problem: **Herpes in Pregnancy**

The Facts:

In our society, it is common for people who have herpes to feel like they have leprosy. Ironically, the majority of the sexually active population has been exposed to herpes—whether or not they have herpes lesions. In other words, having herpes doesn't mean very much these days, as there are very few people an adult can newly infect.

The exception to this is pregnancy. If, at the time she is going into labor, a pregnant woman has an *active* herpes lesion or the sensation that one is coming on, her emerging baby could come into contact with the herpes virus on the way out of the vaginal canal, leading to severe consequences.

What You Can Do:

- Speak to your partner about her herpes infection—try to destigmatize it by discussing how common it is. Insist that she alert her physician.

- Reassure your partner that the presence of herpes lesions in the months preceding the delivery are harmless to the baby.

- Be vigilant around the time of your partner's labor and delivery. If she develops lesions or indicates that she feels the sensation of developing lesions, use a flashlight to help her confirm this and promptly alert her physician.

When to Get More Help:

If your partner is in labor, early labor or has broken her bag of water and develops lesions or the sensation of developing lesions, immediately alert your partner's physician.

8 MONITORING SPECIFIC CONDITIONS

The Problem: **Monitoring "Normal" Baby Movements**

The Facts:

Despite all of the technology used by your partner's physician, you and your partner are in the best position to monitor your baby's daily well-being by simply becoming more aware of your baby's movements. In fact, keeping track of fetal movements can be a wonderful way for you, your partner and the baby to "communicate" prior to the birth. What's "normal"?

FIRST TRIMESTER: Your partner should feel no kicking or movement in the first trimester.

SECOND AND THIRD TRIMESTERS: Beginning around the 20th week of pregnancy, your partner should begin to feel the baby moving and kicking. By the 24th week, healthy babies develop a "routine" for moving and resting. Generally, a baby will move and kick for 20 to 30 minutes and then rest for another 20 to 30 minutes. This regular rhythm of rest and movement is a strong indicator of the well-being of the child, and should remain constant throughout the pregnancy.

On the other hand, the baby is likely to respond to his or her immediate environment and the world outside of the womb through movement. For example, loud noises and your partner's consumption of food are likely to increase the baby's activity, whereas your partner's increased activity may decrease the baby's activity.

You and your partner's ability to feel movement may depend on the baby's position. If the baby's back is parallel to your partner's back, she will feel its movement more clearly than if it is facing your partner's spine, or if the placenta is above the uterus.

What You Can Do:

Apart from making proper monitoring more likely, turning the daily monitoring of the baby's movements into a *joint* activity will make you *look* and feel more involved in your partner's daily experience:

◌ Give your partner a second trimester gift: a simple diary or other journal in which she will record the baby's daily movements, known as a "Kick Journal." Alternatively, she can record the baby's movements on her personal calendar or computer.

◌ Twice each day, after she has eaten—in the morning, during her lunch break or in the evening—encourage her to sit back, relax and focus on the rhythm of the baby's movement for 20 to 30 minutes. One way to do this is to count the number of kicks during this period of time. Ask her to record the rhythm of the baby's movements in her Kick Journal twice per day. This will serve as a great tool for her physician in monitoring the well-being of the baby throughout the pregnancy.

◌ While most people claim not to have the time, your partner will welcome her kick-counting break if you build it into your time together or encourage her to see it as a necessary stress-reducing break in her day—her time alone with you and the baby.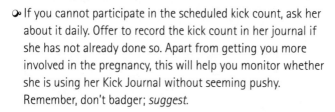

◌ Take the opportunity to participate in the kick-counting rituals as often as possible. You can feel the kicking of the baby by positioning your hands over the area where your partner tells you that she feels the baby the strongest. Ask your partner to position your hands for you.

◌ If you cannot participate in the scheduled kick count, ask her about it daily. Offer to record the kick count in her journal if she has not already done so. Apart from getting you more involved in the pregnancy, this will help you monitor whether she is using her Kick Journal without seeming pushy. Remember, don't badger; *suggest.*

- Whenever your partner feels that the baby's kick count is slowing down, perform the following test: Give her something to eat or drink, preferably something containing natural sugar. With your hands on each side of her belly, wiggle the baby from side to side. Then, ask her to lie on her side and repeat the kick count. A healthy baby will respond to this test by resuming his or her "normal" movement patterns.

- Around the 20th week of pregnancy, ask your partner to tell her physician that she will be monitoring her baby's movements, and to request that her physician describe the circumstances under which he or she would like to receive a phone call. This will ensure that you and your partner feel confident about picking up the phone.

When to Get More Help:

Generally, if, after the 26th week of pregnancy, the baby's kick count slows and does not respond to the test described above, call your partner's physician. While it is likely to be a false alarm—the baby has changed to a position that makes it more difficult for you and your partner to feel the movement—a slowing of movement should never be ignored.

Recognize that you and your partner's attention to the baby's movements and follow-up could make a big difference when addressed promptly. As such, never hesitate to contact your partner's physician about a slow kick count in the middle of the night. After all, by morning, your opportunity to help the baby may have passed. If you cannot reach your partner's physician, take your partner to the maternity ward of the hospital where she will deliver for fetal monitoring. On any given night, you will find many other couples in the waiting room doing the same.

The Problem: Decreased or Increased Amniotic Fluid

The Facts:

A decrease *(oligohydramnion)* or increase *(polyhydramnion)* in the ideal amount of amniotic fluid is highly problematic and requires correction.

An abnormal increase in amniotic fluid is generally associated with diabetes of pregnancy and a number of potential birth defects. An abnormal decrease in the amount of amniotic fluid may be a sign that the baby is not receiving enough nutrients and has "cut corners" in order to redirect all available food to the development of his or her brain and heart.

What You Can Do:

FOR AN ABNORMAL *INCREASE* IN AMNIOTIC FLUID:

◌ Encourage your partner to diligently monitor her baby's daily movements in a "Kick Journal." See the *Monitoring "Normal" Baby Movements* section of this guidebook (page 142) for more information on this useful tool. If she notices a change in the baby's daily movements—an increase or decrease—contact her physician for monitoring.

◌ If you notice a dramatic increase in the size of your partner's belly, particularly as she nears her due date, contact her physician for monitoring.

◌ If your partner's increase in amniotic fluid is associated with diabetes of pregnancy, see the *Diabetes of Pregnancy or Gestational Diabetes* section of this guidebook (page 153) for additional information.

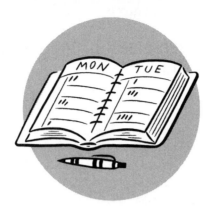

FOR AN ABNORMAL *DECREASE* IN AMNIOTIC FLUID:

❍ If you notice a decrease in the size of your partner's belly at any time in the pregnancy, contact her physician's office for monitoring.

❍ Encourage your partner to diligently monitor her baby's daily movements in a "Kick Journal." See the *Monitoring "Normal" Baby Movements* section of this guidebook (page 142) for more information on this useful tool. If she notices a decrease in the baby's daily movements, contact her physician's office for monitoring.

❍ Ensure that she is supplying the baby with enough nutrients by increasing her protein intake. Compare her diet to the *Ideal Pregnancy Diet* section of this guidebook (page 23).

❍ Suggest that she increase her water consumption to 12 to 14 glasses of water a day.

❍ Encourage her to add sea salt to her food.

❍ Her physician is likely to suggest she take a few days off for bed rest. The ideal resting position is on her side, as lying on her back may cut off blood flow to the baby. During her bed rest, your partner should limit her activity to bathroom trips and visits to the kitchen. If it is not possible for you to spend time with her, arrange for someone to keep her company and provide her with food. See the *Bed Rest Requirements* section of this guidebook (page 89) for more information.

☞ Draw her a *warm* bath. Bath water should not exceed 98 degrees Fahrenheit. Exposure to bath water heated above 98 degrees Fahrenheit may increase the rate of birth defects and, in advanced pregnancy, may lead to premature contractions and delivery. Help her climb in and immerse herself up to her neck. Keep her company or stay close by, as she is likely to require a bathroom trip every 15 to 20 minutes, and will need your help for a safe exit and reimmersion. Spending time in water is an excellent way to increase her amniotic fluid.

When to Get More Help:

Both of these conditions require monitoring by her physician.

In between monitoring appointments, encourage your partner to be especially diligent about keeping her Kick Journal. If she feels a change in the baby's daily movements, consult her physician.

The Problem: **Slow Baby Growth**

The Facts:

Regardless of *your* height or weight, all babies are expected to develop at about the same rate.

If your baby is growing too slowly, it is likely that your partner isn't eating enough, or that she is too active for the amount of food she consumes. In other words, there isn't enough food left over for the baby's growth.

Alternatively, your partner may be eating enough, but the nutrients may be unable to penetrate the placenta and get to the baby.

In situations where the baby is not receiving enough food, there is likely to be a decrease in the baby's growth rate and a decrease in the amount of amniotic fluid produced by the baby.

The good news is that developing babies are very resourceful. At the first sign of nutritional deficiency, babies divert all food to the organs that require food the most, particularly the brain and heart.

What You Can Do:

Your partner's physician is likely to recommend bed rest and increased protein in your partner's diet. In addition, you can do the following to help:

- See the recommendations in the *Decreased or Increased Amniotic Fluid* section of this guidebook (page 145).

- See recommendations in the *Bed Rest Requirements* section of this guidebook (page 89).

- Encourage your partner to consume at least 80 grams of protein per day, and plenty of fresh fruits and vegetables.

- If she cannot keep food down due to nausea or morning sickness—rare after the 14th week of pregnancy—see the recommendations in the *Morning Sickness* section of this guidebook (page 18).

- Make a protein smoothie or a bowl of rich vegetable soup. See the *Quick Protein Smoothie* (page 199) and *Easy Vegetable Soup* (page 200) recipes in the appendix of this guidebook.

- Help her relax with a stress-reducing massage. Remember that pregnant women should lie on their sides if no "pregnancy massage pillow" is available.

- Encourage her to visualize the proper growth of the baby. Ask her to lie down on her side and close her eyes, as you describe how well the baby's various parts are growing. See the *Ideal Baby Growth Chart* in the appendix of this guidebook (page 188) for more information.

- Monitor the well-being of your baby by helping your partner keep up with her "Kick Journal" of the baby's movements. For more information, see the *Monitoring "Normal" Baby Movements* section of this guidebook (page 142).

When to Get More Help:

If you believe your partner is not eating enough, is too active or that the baby is growing too slowly, always address these concerns with your partner's physician. Recognize that this is the time to utilize as many of her physician's suggestions as possible. Full cooperation and communication between you, your partner and her physician can make a tremendous difference to your baby.

A less common reason for slow baby growth is the development of structural problems. If the baby's growth rate does not respond to the suggestions described above, suggest that your partner have an ultrasound examination by a *perinatologist,* a subspecialist in the field of detecting birth defects by ultrasound. This will help you rule out birth defects as the reason for the baby's slow growth.

Sometimes, in spite of good eating habits, nutrients are not able to penetrate the placenta. This condition is most common in women with a variety of diseases, including high blood pressure, lupus and other conditions. If your partner has a preexisting medical condition of any kind, encourage her to *remind* her physician so that the appropriate response can be coordinated.

The Problem: **Fast Baby Growth & Large Babies**

The Facts:

On average, today's babies are born bigger than a generation ago. This increase in baby size does not correlate with an increase in the size of human beings. The question is, are we better off with bigger babies? Not really.

A bigger baby generally means that your partner will have a less mobile pregnancy, a longer labor, more physical trauma to the pelvis, vagina, connective tissue and nerves and an increased chance of requiring a *cesarean section (C-section)*.

What Can You Do:

If her physician has indicated that your baby is growing more quickly than is usual, consider the following:

- ⌖ Remind your partner that she needn't "eat for two." Aside from being a common misconception, most of us already eat for two prior to pregnancy—with the majority of calories consumed being empty calories.

- ⌖ Encourage your partner to eliminate processed carbohydrates (i.e., breads and starch) from her diet. See the *Diabetes of Pregnancy* (page 153) and *Ideal Pregnancy Diet* (page 23) sections of this guidebook for more information.

- ⌖ Help her increase her activity. Invite her on slow, romantic walks—even if it's just window-shopping at the mall.

- ⌖ DO NOT become obsessed with her weight and do not allow her to obsess. Aside from this obsession being destructive to your life together as lovers, pregnancy is not the time to diet or miss a meal.

○ If, despite a modest diet, your partner's pregnancy looks like it's growing very quickly, ask her physician to check her level of amniotic fluid. Often, what looks like a large baby may simply be a rapid accumulation or overproduction of this fluid, also known as *polyhydramnion.* This condition is often associated with shortness of breath, premature labor, diabetes of pregnancy and specific birth defects, which must be addressed by a physician. For more information, see the *Decreased or Increased Amniotic Fluid* section of this guidebook (page 145).

When to Get More Help:

If your partner has been diagnosed with *polyhydramnion,* a condition in which the baby produces too much amniotic fluid, ask your partner's physician to refer you to a *perinatologist,* a subspecialist who is better able to identify and diagnose birth defects by ultrasound.

The Problem: **Diabetes of Pregnancy or Gestational Diabetes**

The Facts:

Diabetes of pregnancy is not the same as the diabetes that generally afflicts adults and children. In fact, as the name suggests, the condition only affects your partner for the term of her pregnancy.

What is it?

Due to her pregnancy, the insulin your partner's body normally produces to process blood sugar becomes less efficient. The result is that her blood sugar—and the baby's—is higher than it should be.

The good news is that most women are able to control this condition by changing their diets—by limiting sugar, starches and carbohydrates and eating more protein—and only a small percentage of women require the use of insulin during their pregnancies.

Your physician will test for this condition between her 24th to 28th weeks of pregnancy.

? Is she relatively overweight, hypoglycemic or does she have low blood sugar? If she "passes" her gestational diabetes test with a score of 125 or higher, ask her physician to test her *fasting insulin level.* If her fasting insulin level is above 15, she may also benefit from a diet designed for women with gestational diabetes. Often women with this fasting insulin level do not efficiently metabolize the carbohydrates they eat and could benefit from the dietary restrictions described below.

What You Can Do:

◦ Once your partner has been diagnosed with diabetes of pregnancy, she'll be sent "back to school," where she will be taught the dos and don'ts of gestational diabetes nutrition. Schedules permitting, try to accompany her to this short class. You may both be surprised to learn that controlling blood "sugar" also requires her to control the consumption of breads, pastas, cereals, crackers, potatoes and some legumes, fruits and vegetables.

○ The following diet suggestions for gestational diabetes, women with hypoglycemia or women with insulin levels over 15 are more strict than generally recommended by physicians, but have been shown to nearly eliminate the need for these women to begin insulin treatment:

THE DOS:

○ The ideal diet is very restrictive with carbohydrates, high in protein and "average" in fat intake. It is similar to *The Zone* or *Atkins* diets, with slight variations.

○ Encourage her to consume 80 grams of protein per day. Meat, fish, milk and cheese, eggs, soybeans and lentils, tofu or protein powder are all acceptable protein sources.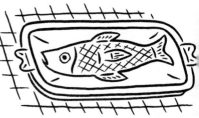

○ She may consume as many servings of vegetables as she would like, so long as the vegetables are not listed as a "starch" in "The Don'ts."

○ Encourage her to limit her consumption of fruit to two portions a day. A reasonable portion of fruit equals a six-ounce cup of berries, cherries or peaches or a single green apple, small orange or half a grapefruit.

○ She may eat as many raw or dry roasted nuts and seeds as she would like (salted or unsalted), so long as they are not roasted in oil.

- Encourage her to increase her consumption of "good fats" and decrease her consumption of "bad fats." Visit your health food store for a variety of "good fat" sources, including *gamma linolenic acid,* found in *evening primrose oil* capsules, 125 milligrams daily, or EPA and DHA fish oil capsules, 1500 miligrams daily. To decrease her consumption of "bad fat," encourage her to choose foods sautéed or stir-fried with butter, olive oil and canola oil and limit her consumption of saturated fat, fried foods, margarine, hydrogenated or partially hydrogenated oil and vegetable shortening.

- Encourage her to drink 8 to 12 glasses of water per day.

THE DON'TS:

- All processed carbohydrates should be eliminated. Processed carbohydrates include bread, pasta, cereal, grain, cookies, rice, beans (except for soy and lentils), crackers, rice cakes, cakes, sugar, honey and candies.

- All starches should be eliminated. Starches include potatoes, sweet potatoes, corn, beets and carrots. Onions and tomatoes may be eaten in limited quantities.

- Fresh or dried fruits and juices are limited to the portions outlined above.

HELPFUL HINTS:

- In the first two weeks of her new diet, she is likely to experience tremendous cravings for carbohydrates and starch. Help her get through this time by picking up any one of the many protein bars on the market with a "40-30-30" balance of carbohydrates, protein and fats. These bars work very well for women with gestational diabetes diet restrictions and should provide her with a "fix" until the cravings subside. Suggest that she eat one-third of a bar between meals.

- Visit your local health food store for *alpha lipoic acid* and *chromium picolinate*, two natural supplements that will help your partner balance her sugar levels. Suggest that she take 200 milliliters of lipoic acid and 200 micrograms of chromium picolinate, three times daily.

- Does she miss her ice cream splurges? Consider bringing home an inexpensive ice cream maker and make homemade ice cream with *stevia*, a natural sweetener available at your local health food store.

- Make yourself available by telephone. Encourage her to call you when her cravings are strong. Talk her through the frustration. Alternatively, suggest that she eat a better food as you talk her through the sensation of eating her favorite candy bar. This really helps!

? And if she slips? Realize that she can only do as much as she can do, and that one or two cookies will not make a big difference, so long as she returns to her suggested diet.

When to Get More Help:

Although your partner's physician will already be monitoring her blood sugar levels, be mindful of whether she is maintaining her recommended diet. If it is clear that she is not, skip the guilt. Instead, encourage her to speak to her physician about her limitations. He or she will determine whether a temporary insulin treatment is appropriate.

The Problem: Low Blood Sugar or Hypoglycemia

The Facts:

Once your partner conceives, her body undergoes a drastic change in hormone levels when the placenta begins to produce additional hormones. This change may also lead to low blood sugar, or *hypoglycemia*. When blood sugar levels drop beyond a certain point, the human body cannot function and goes into crisis. Symptoms of this condition include dizziness, fatigue, sweating, rapid heartbeat, fogginess and loss of consciousness.

Hypoglycemia in pregnancy is more common in women who experienced sugar imbalances prior to their pregnancy, women who are overweight or who have high carbohydrate/low protein diets.

Of course, low blood sugar is more common and becomes more serious in women who experience morning sickness and nausea in the first trimester.

What You Can Do:

- To help your partner avoid hypoglycemia, encourage her to eat three meals and three snacks per day. Each one of her meals should contain a serving of protein.

- Any time she feels faint in between meals, compare her diet to the nutritional guidelines described in the *Ideal Pregnancy Diet* section of this guidebook (page 23). She may require more nutrients than provided by her current meals and snacks.

- If she continues to feel faint despite following the suggestions outlined in the *Ideal Pregnancy Diet* section, encourage her to snack on fruit or sip juice with pulp every hour between her scheduled meals and snacks. Alternatively, surprise her with a nutritious protein smoothie. See the *Quick Protein Smoothie* recipe in the appendix of this guidebook (page 199) for more information.

◌ Nutritional supplements can also help keep blood sugar levels balanced, including 200 micrograms of *chromium picolinate*, taken three times daily and 200 milligrams of *alpha lipoic acid*, taken three times daily. Look for these supplements at your local health food store.

◌ Low blood sugar may also be a sign of *adrenal* deficiency. Adding a fast-absorbing magnesium, such as *magnesium glycinate, magnesium gluconate, magnesium citrate* or *magnesium aspartate* as directed and 25 milligrams of vitamin B complex once daily can be helpful. Slowly increase the recommended dosage of magnesium every few days. Reduce her dosage if she feels fatigued, experiences muscle weakness or diarrhea.

When to Get More Help:

Hypoglycemia may be an early sign of the development of diabetes of pregnancy. Why? Hypoglycemia is often caused by an overproduction of insulin. The more insulin, the lower the blood sugar. Unfortunately, this often leads to insulin resistance. An inability of the body to respond to the insulin it produces is the cause of diabetes of pregnancy. If your partner experiences repeated symptoms of hypoglycemia and feels better when she eats something sweet, ask her physician to test her for diabetes of pregnancy by measuring her fasting glucose and fasting insulin levels.

The Problem: High Blood Pressure or Preeclampsia

The Facts:

There are two groups who experience high blood pressure during pregnancy:

- ▶ Women with preexisting high blood pressure, which is aggravated during pregnancy

- ▶ Women with previously normal blood pressure that experience an increase in the second and—more commonly—in the third trimester of pregnancy (called *preeclampsia*)

Preeclampsia is characterized by increased blood pressure, water retention and an increase in the amount of protein in the urine. In its most severe form, preeclampsia can also affect the kidneys, liver and the blood coagulation system of the body. It is one of the most serious medical complications during pregnancy. This condition is more likely to develop in very young mothers or relatively older mothers. Malnutrition and protein deficiency may increase the incidents of preeclampsia.

Most cases of preeclampsia progress rapidly and require immediate hospitalization, with no opportunity to try home treatment. Only the mildest forms of both elevation of pre-existing high blood pressure or mild preeclampsia may be given a home treatment trial, consisting in large part of complete bed rest.

The recommendations provided below may help prevent the further development of preeclampsia, and may even help women lower their blood pressure levels.

What You Can Do:

- Strictly follow her physician's advice regarding bed rest. See the *Bed Rest Requirements* section of this guidebook for more information (page 89).

- Follow her physician's advice regarding her salt restrictions. Most physicians will not limit her salt intake.

- Encourage her to eat as much garlic as she can tolerate. See the *Easy Vegetable Soup* recipe in the appendix of this guidebook (page 200) as a suggestion. If she cannot eat raw or cooked garlic, visit your local health food store for garlic capsules.

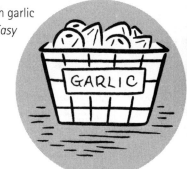

- The juices of dill, cucumber, parsley, dandelion leaf, and onion are helpful for this condition. Consider combining these ingredients into the *Easy Vegetable Soup* recipe in the appendix of this guidebook (page 200).

- Supplement her diet with *magnesium glycinate, magnesium glucante, magnesium citrate, magnesium aspartate* or another fast-absorbing form of magnesium. Use as directed, slowly increasing the dosage every few days. Reduce her dosage if she experiences fatigue, muscle weakness or diarrhea.

- Supplement her diet with 500 milligrams of Coenzyme Q-10 daily, available at your local health food store.

- Other helpful natural supplements include 2000 to 4000 milligrams of vitamin C daily, 800 milligrams of *Mix E* (including vitamins *alpha E, delta E* and *gamma E*) daily, and *lycopene*, 20 to 30 milligrams daily, all found at your local health food store.

When to Get More Help:

If your partner has been prescribed bed rest due to mild high blood pressure, and experiences headache, blurry vision, a significant increase in water retention or pain under her ribs on her right side, call her physician immediately.

The Problem: **Low Thyroid Levels**

The Facts:

The thyroid hormone controls our metabolism and countless other body functions. Symptoms of low thyroid production include:

- cold hands and feet,

- a delay in perspiration,

- fatigue,

- headache,

- leg cramps,

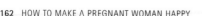

- an inability to "get going" in the morning,

- dry skin,

- brittle nails,

- bags under the eyes,

- easy weight gain, and

- yellow or slightly orange skin when she eats large quantities of carrots.

More importantly, in pregnancy, low thyroid levels are associated with slow fetal brain development. For this reason it is to your advantage to ensure that your partner's thyroid function is performing at *optimal* levels, rather than simply on the low side of "normal."

What You Can Do:

➤ Speak with your partner about the symptoms of low thyroid, particularly the first two listed above. If she feels that these symptoms apply to her, ask her physician to test her thyroid levels.

◌ Recognize that the most common blood test for identifying low thyroid levels, the *thyroid stimulated hormone* test (TSH), fails to diagnose the majority of people who experience the symptoms listed above.

◌ Instead, ask her physician to test her *T3 Free* and *T4 Free* levels. These tests monitor the *active* thyroid hormone, itself.

◌ If her *T3 Free* and *T4 Free* levels are low, or on the low side of "normal," urge her physician to provide her with *natural* thyroid supplements. Remember, you want her level optimal during her pregnancy.

When to Get More Help:

Whenever she displays symptoms associated with low thyroid, always consult her physician and request that she be tested.

When beginning thyroid therapy, it is necessary to slowly build up the dosage. Your partner will immediately know when she has increased her dosage beyond what her body requires when she feels irritable, shaky, sweats easily or feels her heart pounding. If this occurs, encourage her to reduce her dosage and consult with her physician.

The Problem: Vaginal Bleeding in the First Trimester

(Also see the *Vaginal Bleeding in the Second & Third Trimesters* section of this guidebook [page 166].)

The Facts:

The most common reason for vaginal bleeding in the first trimester is actual or threatened miscarriage. Unfortunately, a significant number of pregnancies don't "hold," and will be naturally miscarried, either because the fetus is genetically unfit or for any number of other reasons.

Despite this, realize that vaginal bleeding does not always mean your partner has lost the pregnancy.

Bleeding can also be a sign of an *ectopic* pregnancy, a pregnancy that has implanted outside of the uterus, which can be dangerous if not diagnosed early. Ectopic pregnancies are characterized by increasing pain and swelling of the abdomen in the first few months of the pregnancy.

Additionally, many women bleed during the first trimester due to a deficiency of the hormone *progesterone.* A small percentage of women may also experience light menstrual bleeding—and less commonly, a normal menstrual cycle—in the first few months of the pregnancy.

What You Can Do:

◑ **Threatened or actual miscarriage.** Any time your partner bleeds heavily, call her physician. When she goes in, request an ultrasound to determine the baby's condition.

If she is miscarrying, she may nonetheless require medical attention. Often, women who miscarry bleed very heavily and require medical attention to accelerate the process and avoid hemorrhaging. Be sure to give her physician information about how long she has been bleeding and whether she is experiencing cramping.

Visit your health food store for *arnica,* a homeopathic remedy, and *Maca Maca* capsules or powder. Both of these natural remedies have been known to preserve pregnancies threatened by miscarriage.

○ **Symptoms of ectopic pregnancy.** Any time she experiences abdominal pain or swelling, vaginal bleeding, shoulder pain, dizziness or a clammy feeling, call her physician. Ectopic pregnancies can become life-threatening to the mother if treatment is delayed.

○ **Low progesterone.** Encourage your partner's physician to measure her *progesterone* level. Progesterone levels under 20 should be supplemented with natural progesterone.

When to Get More Help:

Any time your partner bleeds during the first trimester, contact her physician and insist that she be seen immediately if the bleeding is heavy or if the bleeding is accompanied by pain. In the meantime, make note of as many of her symptoms as possible.

During your visit, ask your partner's physician to outline what to do and under what circumstances to call if bleeding resumes or increases.

The Problem: Vaginal Bleeding in the Second & Third Trimesters

(Also see the *Vaginal Bleeding in the First Trimester* section of this guidebook [page 164].)

The Facts:

While less frequent, bleeding in the second and third trimesters often happens as a result of *placenta previa,* when the *placenta* sits over or too close to the cervix.

Alternatively, light bleeding, pain and cramping can be a sign of an *abruption of the placenta,* a life-threatening condition where your partner bleeds behind the placenta.

Bleeding and a feeling of pressure can be the first sign of a premature delivery due to a weak *cervix* that cannot hold the pregnancy.

Finally, it is common for pregnant women to bleed after intercourse. Usually this is of no significance, but should always be reported, as this may be the first sign of a placenta that has implanted to closely to the cervix.

What You Can Do:

ᐁ Always bring bleeding to the attention of her physician.

ᐁ Make note of whether she is experiencing bleeding, pressure, cramps or any other symptoms you regard as abnormal to her pregnancy. A combination of bleeding and pain or bleeding, cramping and pressure should be reported immediately.

ᐁ Your ability to describe the situation will be helpful, as your partner may not be in a position to describe her symptoms.

When to Get More Help:

Always report bleeding in the second and third trimester as soon as possible.

After evaluation, ask your partner's physician to describe the circumstances requiring another call.

The Problem: **Multiple Pregnancies (i.e., Twins, Triplets, etc.)**

The Facts:

Despite the fact that the human uterus is not designed to grow more than one baby at a time and that very few twin pregnancies make it to full term, with today's higher frequency of *in vitro fertilization* (IVF) and egg donation, many more women find themselves pregnant with multiples than ever before. This creates a variety of complications for the pregnancy, including:

- higher incidence of premature labor,

- situations in which one or more fetuses are not receiving enough nutrients and their growth slows,

- higher incidence of cervical weakness *(cervical incompetence),*

- higher incidence of bladder infections, and

- higher incidence of blood pressure problems.

In short, multiple pregnancies are always considered "high risk" pregnancies and should be monitored closely.

What You Can Do:

- Discourage your partner from eating for two, three or more. Suggest that she slightly increase the amount of protein she eats to 90 grams per day and the amount of water she drinks to 10 to 14 glasses per day.

- While single-fetus pregnancies allow a woman to step up her physical activity without compromising the baby's develop-ment, this is not the case with multiple pregnancies. Even physical fitness professionals must reduce their activity for the well-being of their multiple pregnancy.

- Even if her physician has checked the condition of your partner's cervix and given it a clean bill of health, encourage her to rest on her side as often as possible. The measurement of the cervix by pelvic ultrasound should be conducted every two weeks, from the 16th to the 32nd week of the pregnancy.

- Apply all the suggestions related to preventing premature labor. Encourage her to become aware of the activity of her uterus (i.e., contractions). See the *Premature Labor* section of this guidebook (page 175) for more information.

- If she has been put on bed rest, help her stay off of her feet using the information provided in the *Bed Rest Requirements* section of this guidebook (page 89).

- If you learn that one of the fetuses is growing more quickly than the others, speak with her physician about whether your partner is a candidate for one of the new laser procedures available for this condition. These procedures use laser treatments to redirect blood flow in the placenta to ensure that underfed fetuses receive their share of nutrients.

- Studies have shown that multiple pregnancies in excess of three fetuses have a significantly higher rate of very early premature delivery that may lead to cerebral palsy and mental retardation in all of the fetuses. Some patients elect to selectively reduce the number to ensure the health of the remaining fetuses. There is a push by some medical professionals to reduce all triple pregnancies to twins; however, there is not sufficient data to support this. Simply following proper preventive guidelines in triple pregnancy is likely to result in as good of an outcome as twin births.

○ If a "normal" pregnancy creates physiological and physical changes that are hard to cope with, a multiple pregnancy enhances all of these difficulties. This is when you can be the most helpful to your partner. Even if she is not complaining, recognize that, despite her enthusiasm, a multiple pregnancy is hard work. Help her minimize her workload. Solicit and accept offers of help from family and friends where needed.

When to Get More Help:

Multiple pregnancies are prone to premature labor and weakening of the cervix throughout the pregnancy. Alert her physician if your partner reports unusual, more frequent contractions or the symptoms associated with cervical weakness. See the *Cervical Weakness* section of this guidebook (page 178) for more information.

9 PREPARING FOR DELIVERY

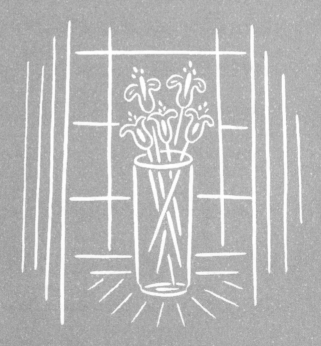

The Problem: **False Contractions or Braxton Hicks**

The Facts:

It is common for women to experience labor contractions throughout pregnancy. If these contractions do not lead to actual labor, they are labeled "false" contractions, or "Braxton Hicks," after the doctor who first described them. As your partner's pregnancy develops she is likely to notice these contractions more often.

The good news is that contractions that do not lead to premature labor are otherwise harmless. Once her physician evaluates the contractions and verifies that they have not affected the cervix, your partner will be sent home.

Unfortunately, a minority of women feel false contractions more strongly. Often these contractions disturb their sleep and physical activity.

What You Can Do:

To lessen the occurrence of painful or otherwise distracting false contractions:

- Encourage your partner to stay well-hydrated by drinking 8 to 12 glasses of water per day.

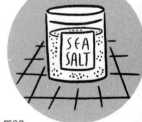

- Suggest that she add sea salt to her food in order to replace the sodium and potassium that her body loses through perspiration.

- Replace her calcium supplements with magnesium supplements. Calcium causes the uterine muscles to *contract* while magnesium encourages these muscles to *relax*.

Visit your local health food store for *magnesium glycinate, magnesium gluconate, magnesium citrate, magnesium aspartate* or another fast-absorbing magnesium. Encourage her to take the suggested dosage with food, and slowly increase the dosage every few days until she begins to feel sleepy or experiences more than two soft bowel movements per day. Reduce her dosage if she experiences fatigue, muscle weakness or diarrhea.

- Encourage her to increase her consumption of "good fats" and decrease her consumption of "bad fats." This change will help decrease her contractions. Visit your health food store for a variety of "good fat" sources, including *gamma linolenic acid,* found in *evening primrose oil* capsules, 125 milligrams daily, or EPA and DHA fish oil capsules, 1500 milligrams daily. To decrease her consumption of "bad fat," encourage your partner to choose foods sautéed or stir-fried with butter, olive oil and canola oil, and limit her consumption of saturated fat, fried foods, margarine, hydrogenated or partially hydrogenated oil and vegetable shortening.

- Suggest that she decrease the activities that enhance her false contractions. Discourage her from exercising to the point when contractions occur. This is a signal that she is being too active. Alternatively, suggest that she replace her usual exercise routine with a water activity.

- Draw her a *warm* bath. Bath water should not exceed 98 degrees Fahrenheit. Exposure to bath water heated above 98 degrees Fahrenheit may increase the rate of birth defects and, in advanced pregnancy, may lead to premature contractions and delivery. Help her climb in and immerse herself up to her neck. Keep her company or stay close by, as she is likely to require a bathroom trip every 15 to 20 minutes, and will need your help for a safe exit and reimmersion. This will decrease uterine activity and premature contractions.

When to Get More Help:

Always bring initial contractions to the attention of her physician. He or she will determine whether these sensations are "false" or the real thing.

Once your partner begins to experience false contractions, ask her physician to describe the specific symptoms that will require you to contact him or her again.

The Problem: **Premature Labor**

The Facts:

Premature labor is one of the most complicated, costly and potentially devastating conditions in pregnancy.

Thirty years ago, when doctors first attempted to control this problem and discovered that alcohol consumption postponed the onset of labor, they went so far as to hook pregnant women up to *intravenous* bags filled with alcohol. Just imagine what it must have been like to walk through a maternity ward filled with intoxicated pregnant women. Happily, this experiment didn't last long and produced only minimal benefits. Yet even today, the most sophisticated modern techniques cannot significantly improve on this.

The best evidence suggests that good nutrition and the vigilance of the mother-to-be is the best defense against premature labor.

What You Can Do:

- If she is having contractions and believes that she is going into premature labor—even while lying on a hospital bed and receiving treatment—encourage her to lie on her side and use her *mind* and *willpower* to control the contractions. Believe it or not, this can be extremely helpful. Encourage her to visualize that her contractions are subsiding, and that her cervix is closing. Ask her to breathe deeply and imagine that her labor is fading away as she floats on a calm body of water. Suggest that she repeat to herself: *"I am relaxed, my muscles are relaxed and my uterus is relaxed."* The simple act of relaxing her muscles is likely to reduce her contractions, but the mental focus on ending premature labor has helped many women avoid the onset.

- Encourage her to stay well hydrated by drinking 8 to 12 glasses of water per day.

- Suggest that she add sea salt to her food to replace the sodium and potassium that her body loses through perspiration.

- Replace her calcium supplements with magnesium supplements. Calcium causes the uterine muscles to *contract* while magnesium encourages these muscles to *relax.* Visit your local health food store for *magnesium glycinate, magnesium gluconate, magnesium citrate, magnesium aspartate* or another fast-absorbing magnesium. Encourage her to take the suggested dosage with food, and slowly increase the dosage every few days until she begins to feel sleepy or experiences more than two soft bowel movements per day. Reduce her dosage if she experiences fatigue, muscle weakness or diarrhea.

- Encourage her to increase her consumption of "good fats" and decrease her consumption of "bad fats." Visit your health food store for a variety of "good fat" sources, including *gamma linolenic acid,* an active ingredient in *evening primrose oil* capsules, 125 milligrams daily, or EPA and DHA fish oil capsules, 1500 milligrams daily. To decrease her consumption of "bad fat," encourage your partner to choose foods sautéed or stir-fried with butter, olive oil and canola oil, and limit her consumption of saturated fat, fried foods, margarine, hydrogenated or partially hydrogenated oil and vegetable shortening.

- If she has been assigned to bed rest, avoiding premature labor depends entirely on following this advice. Do everything you can to make her bed rest possible. See the *Bed Rest Requirements* section of this guidebook (page 89) for more information.

- Suggest that she also decrease the activities that enhance her false contractions. Discourage her from exercising to the point when contractions occur—this is a signal that she is being too active. Alternatively, suggest that she replace her usual exercise routine with a water activity.

○ Draw her a *warm* bath. Exposure to bath water heated above 98 degrees Fahrenheit may increase the rate of birth defects and, in advanced pregnancy, may lead to premature contractions and delivery. Help her climb in and immerse herself up to her neck. Keep her company or stay close by, as she is likely to require a bathroom trip every 15 to 20 minutes, and will need your help for a safe exit and reimmersion. This will decrease uterine activity.

○ Inquire whether she was given a routine bladder infection test in her second trimester; this will prevent premature labor due to "silent" bladder infections. See the *Urinary Tract & Bladder Infections* section of this guidebook (page 131) for more information.

○ Vaginal infection may cause premature labor. If your partner is at high risk for, or experiencing, premature labor, encourage her to visit her physician for routine vaginal cultures.

○ Encourage her to consult her physician regarding cervical weakness. See the *Cervical Weakness* section of this guidebook (page 178) for more information.

○ Above all, encourage your partner to *relax*. A stressful professional life or concern about the baby *docs* affect the timing of labor. Worrying can cause an increase in the uterine contractions that could lead to premature labor. Help her control her level of daily stress. Simply teaching her how to relax will reduce the incidence of premature contractions.

When to Get More Help:

Alert her physician any time her premature contractions don't end relatively soon after she stops to rest and relax.

Always ask her physician to describe the symptoms that he or she believes require an immediate follow-up phone call.

The Problem: **Cervical Weakness**

The Facts:

Although most people associate premature labor with early contractions, a weak cervix incapable of "holding" the pregnancy *(cervical incompetence)* is another major culprit of premature labor, particularly in the second trimester. Unfortunately, symptoms of a weak cervix are generally mild and only become apparent once the damage is irreversible. For this reason, the best way to avoid premature labor by a weak cervix is to recognize whether your partner is a likely candidate and work to prevent the weakening.

Who is likely to develop a weak cervix?

▶ Women who have terminated pregnancies in the past.

▶ Women whose mothers used DES, a drug prescribed in the 1940s, in the Southern United States, to avoid premature delivery. DES may cause the daughters of these women to develop weak cervixes.

▶ Women who have undergone procedures called *LEEP* or *LEEP cone biopsy,* in which part of the cervix is removed in the course of precancerous treatment of the cervix.

▶ Women who are pregnant with multiples (i.e., twins, triplets, etc.).

Unfortunately, the development of this condition is not associated with uterine contractions or any other specific symptom. Once the cervix weakens to the point where it begins to open, your partner may feel a persistent pressure in the cervix or lower pelvis, the top of the uterus may drop so that her belly will appear smaller and there may be an increase in vaginal discharge that may include mucous with spots of blood. It is also possible for a weak cervix to open without any of these symptoms.

What You Can Do:

- Make your partner aware of the groups of women at risk for developing a weak cervix. Encourage her to alert her physician if she believes she is at risk.

- Encourage her to request that her physician use an ultrasound to check her cervix throughout the pregnancy. Normal pelvic exams won't properly diagnose this condition because the weakening of the cervix occurs on the *inside* of the cervix. The cervix should be examined every few weeks, from the 16th to the 32nd week of the pregnancy.

- Once a weak cervix has been diagnosed, she will likely be assigned to strict bed rest or prescribed a surgical procedure determined by the degree of weakness and her stage of pregnancy. Make it more likely that she will heed her physician's advice by making arrangements that will allow for her to be in bed. For more information see the *Bed Rest Requirements* section of this guidebook (page 89).

- If she has no problems with her cervix in one pregnancy, she is unlikely to have problems in subsequent pregnancies.

When to Get More Help:

Cervical weakness always requires the monitoring of a physician. Contact her physician in between visits if your partner is in a high risk group and feels that her uterus has "dropped," feels an increase of pressure or observes an increase in vaginal discharge.

The Problem: **Where to Deliver**

The Facts:

In many books and pamphlets on labor and delivery, home births and hospitals are often given equal billing. In spite of this and the "home birth revolution" of the last 30 years, the overwhelming majority of parents choose to deliver their children in hospital facilities.

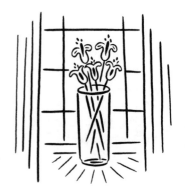

Why is this?

First, the labor and delivery departments of most hospitals have changed radically in the last 30 years. Where it used to be that women had very little freedom in choosing how their children would be delivered, today's hospitals have softened their delivery environments and regularly give their customers a variety of choices about levels of intervention, medication, participation of family members and contact with the newborn. That's right: "customers." Today's hospitals recognize that women and their partners have a choice, and go to great lengths to "earn" each family's health-care dollars.

The second reason most couples opt for hospital deliveries is safety. Assuming an ideal, complication-free birth, home deliveries would be a great alternative. Unfortunately, in many cases the lowest-risk pregnancy has been known to become a high-risk delivery in a matter of minutes. While hospitals are equipped to immediately respond to a life-threatening event, a home birth necessarily delays treatment while the mother, baby or both are transferred to a nearby hospital. These minutes or hours can make a tremendous difference in the mother and baby's chances for a positive outcome.

A related third option is the "birthing center," where doctors, midwives or other attendants assist in the delivery of the baby in a homelike setting. Unfortunately, unless the birthing center is fully integrated into the labor and delivery department of a hospital, it shares all of the disadvantages of a home birth—with two additions: You're *not* at home, *and* the bed your partner delivers in may be just as "overused" as any hospital bed.

What You Can Do:

Discuss the various delivery options with your pregnant partner and her physician. The choice is a personal one, but may be determined for you based on the medical realities of the pregnancy and your own level of risk tolerance.

CHOOSING A HOSPITAL:

- ◌ Exercise your consumer power by shopping around for the facility that best meets your needs. Often doctors have attendance privileges at several local hospitals and choose the delivery hospital for their patients. Find out what options are available to you in order to determine where you and your partner will be most comfortable.

- ◌ Ideally, you want your hospital to meet the following two criteria:

  - ▶ A facility that allows your partner to be delivered by her physician of choice

  - ▶ A facility that has obstetric anesthesia, a high-risk obstetric specialist and pediatric intensive care—all available 24 hours a day

? Why is 24-hour obstetric anesthesia necessary? In the event that your partner requires an emergency *cesarean section (C-section)* or epidural pain relief, the presence of a designated anesthesiologist will ensure that she receives this care without delay.

? Why is a 24-hour high-risk obstetric specialist desirable? The presence of this specialist will give your delivering physician the opportunity to receive a second opinion about various complications that may arise in labor.

? Why is a 24-hour pediatric intensive care unit necessary? This unit will provide immediate professional care for unexpected complications in labor that require immediate attention for premature and full-term babies alike.

? Why is it important to have as many of these components as possible in your hospital? A hospital that does not have these services available around the clock will require the mother or child in trouble to wait or to be transferred to another facility—and the required care to be necessarily delayed.

! On the other hand, realize that many smaller and suburban hospitals that may not have doctors who are specialists in these fields available 24 hours a day have designed functional ways of providing these services to their patients on a 24-hour basis. Ask her physician about these services.

- A private teaching hospital that also grants privileges to private physicians is a great option. Doctors working in teaching hospitals are often exposed to the latest medical information and work with the best equipment.

- Public teaching hospitals may be your most economical choice. While these hospitals are usually the least luxurious, and your partner will not have a private physician, she will receive an excellent quality of care that includes all of the services described above.

? What if you live in a rural area? While rural hospitals may not have the 24-hour facilities described above, they do give you and your partner an opportunity to deliver close

to home, with a physician you know and trust. Moreover, most rural hospitals have a very efficient system
for quickly transporting a high-risk patient and providing
support along the way. Ask her physician about these
services.

OTHER DELIVERIES:

❧ If you choose to deliver at home or at a birthing center, check
the qualifications of the birthing assistant or midwife you will
use. It is crucial for this service provider to be licensed by the
state or province in which you live, *regardless* of the glowing
references of the last couple who used her. They may not have
had the complications your delivery will face.

❧ Verify what your backup plan will be for transferring your
partner and baby to a medical center that can respond to
complications. Make sure that this hospital can provide a
team to immediately perform an emergency *cesarean section
(C-section)* if needed, at any hour of the day or night.

When to Get More Help:

Still confused after speaking with her physician? Contact the
hospital(s) where her physician has attendance privileges. Every
hospital has maternity department coordinators whose job
focuses on providing information to couples who are considering
delivering in (i.e., bringing their business to) that particular
hospital. Take a tour, read through the information packets provided and inquire whether the hospital can meet your and your
partner's needs. Ideally, stay focused on the standard of care—
and how quickly your partner and the baby can be seen by a subspecialist—rather than the color of the recovery room walls.

The Problem: Delivery Options & "Natural Childbirth"

The Facts:

"Natural childbirth" generally refers to a vaginal delivery that does not make use of pain medication or surgical procedures. Instead, women and their partners study a variety of breathing techniques that help women get through the pain of childbirth. Another component of natural childbirth is that the baby remains in the mother's room following the delivery, rather than in the hospital nursery.

There was a time when women felt that they had to make a definitive choice between a "natural" and conventional delivery. Why is this? In the past, most hospital deliveries where strict— women were brought in, medicated and delivered while they were still unconscious or heavily sedated. Their babies would be taken away to the nursery, with very limited opportunities for mother and child to bond during the first few days of life.

This is no longer the case in North American hospitals. These days, hospitals vie for your family's health-care dollars by allowing you to make decisions about pain medication and procedures, who will be invited into the room during delivery and whether your baby sleeps in the room with your partner following delivery.

As a result, many women choose to combine aspects of conventional and natural deliveries, in order to make the experience of childbirth more enjoyable.

What You Can Do:

◌ Encourage your partner to explore her options. In today's more patient-friendly hospital environments, there are no right or wrong choices.

- If she is concerned about the pain of labor, but would like to be clear-minded throughout her delivery, she may choose an epidural, a nerve block which limits the sensation of pain but allows her to be wide awake, pushing and participating throughout the labor.

- Many women like the idea—and the *challenge*—of bringing their child into the world without the help of pain medication or procedure. Perhaps they feel a bit of competitive spirit with those women who describe their natural childbirth triumphs. Discourage her from getting sucked into competition. This is her delivery, and she should do what is right for *her*.

- When considering a pain medication-free delivery, encourage her to speak with her *most open* friends. Some women suffer through hours of assistance-free labor, only to ask for an epidural at the very end. Aside from producing a less pleasant experience, many women report that these eleventh-hour requests make them feel as though they have "failed." This is ironic, when—pain medication or not—they have succeeded in bringing a child into the world. Make it clear to your partner that, regardless of assistance, delivery is a triumph in itself.

- Depending on her level of pain tolerance, hearing stories like the one described above may convince your partner to opt for an epidural at the beginning of her labor. Remind her that there is nothing wrong with choosing a birthing plan that focuses on creating a pleasant experience for you both.

- Regardless of the delivery you plan for, sign up for birthing classes. You will both receive valuable information about the process and what to expect. You will also learn a variety of breathing and pushing exercises, important to know regardless of her plans for medical assistance. After all, the pain relief may not be ready when she is.

- Make a birthing plan. Discuss details such as pain preferences and delivery room guests, so that they can be clearly communicated to her physician and—later—to the nurses in the hospital. Recognize that if your requests are within what is allowed by hospital policy, they will be accommodated. You will find that the hospital nurses will be your strongest advocates in this process.

- Finally, regardless of your plans, recognize that childbirth is unpredictable. Your mother-to-be may plan for a natural delivery and end up requiring a *cesarean section (C-section)*. On the other hand, she may plan on an early epidural and find that her labor is so easy, that she is more comfortable walking off the contractions down the hallway.

When to Get More Help:

Sit and talk to friends and family who have recently gone through the experience of childbirth. Ask them what they would have done differently and what they would do next time. Most of them had specific birthing plans that may have worked out differently than they expected. Encourage your partner to do the same in order to gain a perspective on labor and delivery often not addressed in childbirth books.

APPENDICES

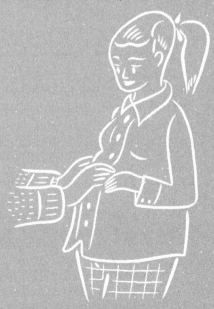

Appendix One:
Ideal Baby Growth Chart

Recognize that doctors measure ideal fetal development in weight, not length. Length measurements from the top of the head to the bottom of the buttocks (known as crown-to-rump measurements, or "CR") are provided to give parents an approximate idea of the size of their developing baby throughout the pregnancy. Recognize that the weights and sizes of healthy babies can vary.

First Trimester

WEEK ONE TO TWO: During the "first" two weeks of pregnancy, your partner is not actually pregnant, as the calculations of pregnancy time only *technically* begin on the 1st day of her last period.

WEEK THREE TO FOUR: Your mother-to-be experiences exaggerated PMS symptoms, due to an egg that has been fertilized by your sperm. Immediately, cells begin multiplying, forming an *embryo*.

WEEK FIVE: Your partner is now one week late with her period. The fertilized egg— now an *embryo*—implants into the lining of the uterus. Cells continue multiplying.

WEEK SIX: Cells multiply in layers now as the heart, brain and skeleton begin to form. The embryo's heartbeat can be heard. Your embryo is less than a quarter of an inch in CR size.

WEEK SEVEN: Your embryo develops lungs, intestines, a liver and eyes, but his or her overall size is still less than half an inch in CR size.

WEEK NINE: Your embryo has become a *fetus* with moving arms and legs.

WEEK ELEVEN: Your fetus grows fingernails.

WEEK THIRTEEN: Your fetus's head becomes rounder as all bones begin forming. Fetal formation is completed, and it measures approximately 2 inches in CR size and weighs less than one ounce.

Second Trimester

WEEK FIFTEEN: Your fetus's ears and eyes move forward to look more like a baby and less like a fish. The fetus measures approximately 4 inches CR and weighs nearly four ounces, and may suck his or her thumb. By now, your physician may be able to identify the sex of your fetus through ultrasound.

WEEK SEVENTEEN: Fat begins to form, as the fetus's measurement climbs to over 4 inches total, or more than 2 inches CR, and between three and four ounces in weight.

WEEK NINETEEN: The uterus may be faintly felt just below the mother's belly button.

WEEK TWENTY-ONE: Your fetus will begin growing hair and may measure approximately 7 inches in CR size and weigh between ten and twelve ounces.

WEEK TWENTY-THREE: Your fetus develops eyelids and eyebrows.

WEEK TWENTY-FIVE: The fetus can now hiccup and hear your voice, and grows to approximately 10 inches CR and a weight of over one pound.

Third Trimester

WEEK TWENTY-SEVEN: Your fetus begins to grow more rapidly.

WEEK TWENTY-NINE: Your fetus can now open and close its eyes, measures over 11 inches CR and may weigh over three pounds.

WEEK THIRTY-ONE: The uterus has risen four inches above the belly button. He or she may shift to a head-down position during this time.

WEEK THIRTY-THREE: Your fetus will grow to 12 inches in CR size and a weight of approximately five pounds in the next week or so.

WEEK THIRTY-FIVE: Your fetus becomes more active: kicking, blinking and continuing to urinate on his or her own.

WEEK THIRTY-SEVEN: Your fetus may measure 20 inches in total length, or 15 inches in CR size, and weigh approximately six pounds.

WEEK THIRTY-NINE: With all organs fully developed, final touches are put in place that may cause your fetus to put on an ounce per day. At the time of delivery, the weight and size of healthy babies can range from six to nine pounds and between 17 and 22 inches in total length.

WEEK FORTY: It's show time, but don't be surprised if he or she makes you wait a couple of extra weeks.

Appendix Two:
Pregnancy Monitoring & Testing Choices

The following list of common tests performed in pregnancy is designed to provide you with more information on each procedure and the information it can provide about your growing baby.

First Trimester Monitoring:

First trimester testing focuses on ruling out birth defects and confirming that the early pregnancy is progressing as it should. Recognize that the reliability of these tests is entirely dependent on properly assessing the *exact* date of conception. Simply miscalculating this date by two or three days can throw off the readings and may require you to wait another week for more helpful information. For this reason, your partner's tests may be repeated before a final diagnosis is made.

○ **Hormone level monitoring.** In the first 10 days following your partner's missed period, the well-being of the new pregnancy will be assessed by monitoring her *estrogen, progesterone* and *Beta HCG* hormone levels. In the first 10 days of pregnancy, the Beta HCG level should double every 48 hours.

○ **Ultrasound.** Additional information about early pregnancy is provided by ultrasound monitoring, a machine that uses sound waves to created images of the pregnancy on a monitor. As early as the 7th or 10th day after your partner's menstrual cycle is late, her physician can already see the pregnancy within the uterus. This early screening can visually verify that the pregnancy is developing as it should and can also determine the number of embryos (i.e., twins, triplets, etc.).

Eighteen days after your partner's menstrual cycle is late, her physician can already see the heartbeat by ultrasound.

- **Blood tests and ultrasound.** At the end of the first trimester, around 10 to 13 weeks, ultrasound will be used again to measure the thickness of the skin on the fetus's neck. This is called a nuchal lucancy test, the accuracy of which has been shown to be close to 98 percent. This, combined with blood testing, provides her physician with information on whether your partner is at a higher risk for producing a child with chromosomal defects than other women in her age group.

- **Chorionic villi sampling (CVS).** If the mother-to-be is at higher risk for producing a child with chromosomal defects, she may be advised to take an additional test, called a *CVS procedure,* in which a small piece of the fetal placenta is collected to learn more about the specific chromosomal composition of your developing baby. This test is performed between the 9th and 11th weeks of pregnancy. CVS should be considered under the following circumstances:

  ▶ Early tests indicate a higher risk for chromosomal defects

  ▶ Family history includes nonchromosomal defects only detected by this procedure

  ▶ When the mother would not consider terminating a pregnancy with birth defect in the second trimester, but would consider doing so in the first

  ▶ When parents are too anxious to wait for second trimester amniocentesis results

The CVS procedure carries a minimal increase in degree of risk over amniocentesis. Ensure that this procedure is performed by a physician who routinely conducts this test, as less familiar hands increase the risk of complications. When in doubt, ask to be referred to a specialist.

- **Genetic counseling.** Once your pregnancy is progressing well, it may be prudent to seek a consultation to rule out common genetic diseases. Who should have genetic counseling?

- Women who have previously delivered genetically abnormal children.

- Men and women with family histories of genetic defects.

- *Ashkenazi* Jews, or Jews of Eastern European descent. This population is prone to a variety of genetic diseases, the best known of which is *Tay-Sachs* disease.

- African Americans. This population exhibits high incidents of *sickle cell anemia.*

- Men and women of Mediterranean origin with a family history of anemia.

- Women who, from a week after conception, were exposed to medication, toxic material, a large amount of alcohol, recreational drugs or other elements known to be harmful to pregnancy.

Speak to her physician for a referral to a geneticist. Every hospital has or is affiliated with a facility that tests for genetic defects. To determine whether you or your pregnant partner fall into a high risk group, it may be necessary to speak with family members and help your partner recall what medications or other substances she was exposed to in the week following conception.

Second Trimester Monitoring:

Second trimester monitoring focuses less on the development of the baby and more on specifically diagnosing physical and chromosomal deformities:

◦ **Triple test.** This test is performed between the 15th and 19th weeks of pregnancy. Initially, the triple test was used to rule out a disease called *spina bifida.* In the last few years, the use of this test has been expanded to determine a pregnant woman's true chances for producing a child with chromosomal defects, by individual probability rather than by her age group.

While not 100 percent accurate, the triple test provides women and their partners with more information about their individual statistical risk, which can help them better decide about more invasive procedures like *amniocentesis*. In the past, this decision was made simply based on whether the mother-to-be was over 35. From a medically conservative perspective, her physician may nonetheless advise a mother-to-be over 35 to proceed with amniocentesis.

- **Amniocentesis.** Amniocentesis testing—where a needle is used to extract a small amount of the amniotic fluid—is the most common procedure used to determine whether your baby has developed chromosomal defects. It is usually performed between the 16th and 20th weeks, but may be performed as early as the 13th week with a slightly higher risk of complications. While amniocentesis carried some risk of complications, this risk is greatly reduced when the procedure is performed by a *perinatologist* or an obstetrician who performs amniocentesis in high volume. In the hands of an experienced physician, the procedure is quick and simple. Following her amniocentesis, your partner will be advised to reduce her activity and engage in limited bed rest for a period of 48 hours. Your partner may not need to have an amniocentesis or a CVS test if her risk factor for producing a child with chromosomal defects, based on her age and other early blood testing, is lower that the risk factor for complications associated with these procedures.

- **Percutaneous umbilical cord blood sampling (PUBS).** If your partner's amniocentesis results indicate that further testing is required to detect potential defects, a *PUBS* procedure will be offered to you between the 18th and 36th weeks of pregnancy. While very similar to the amniocentesis—a needle extracts fluid from a blood vessel in the umbilical cord—the PUBS test is considered to be more accurate, but also carries a higher risk of complications.

- **Structural ultrasound.** At 20 weeks, your baby's body development will be assessed by a *perinatologist,* a doctor specially trained in identifying physical defects by ultrasound. Today's structural ultrasound may assisted by three-dimensional ultrasound technology.

- **Bladder infection culture.** It is common for pregnant women to develop bladder infections even in the absence of common symptoms. For this reason, pregnant women in their second trimesters should be routinely screened for "silent" bladder infections to prevent infection-related complications, including premature labor.

Third Trimester Monitoring:

Testing performed in the third trimester focuses on monitoring the well-being of the baby and ensuring the proper growth and development of the child:

- **Ultrasound.** Third trimester ultrasounds look more closely at how your baby is growing, moving, breathing, hiccupping, emptying his or her bladder and the baby's position in relation to the uterus (i.e., breech, vertex, transverse, etc).

- **Doppler blood flow test.** Your physician may use D*oppler blood flow,* an ultrasound technique that measures blood flow to the baby's specific organs. This technique is usually used in the third trimester to determine whether the baby is receiving enough blood through the placenta. The two most common conditions that require additional testing by way of this procedure are slow baby growth and *preeclampsia.*

- **Fetal heart monitor.** The fetal heart monitor that is the standard of monitoring during labor may also be used during an office visit to asses the well-being of the pregnancy in high risk situations and to verify the onset of labor or premature labor.

Common Foods Pregnant Women Should Avoid

- Raw meats

- Meat not fully cooked

- Uncooked meat leftovers

- Low-grade ground beef

- Raw or unrefrigerated eggs

- Milk or eggs past their due dates

- Unpasteurized milk

- Fish and shellfish that is not fresh

- Raw fish, shellfish or sushi (although pregnant women in Japan eat it without incident)

- Big fish (i.e., tuna and swordfish)

- Excess caffeine (including chocolate, hot chocolate, coffee, tea)

- Large amounts of sugar, including sugar in honey and fruits

- Foods with preservatives and additives, artificial colors and flavors

- Foods that don't smell or taste right to the mother-to-be

Appendix Four:

Common Activities Pregnant Women Should Avoid

- Lying flat on her abdomen after the first trimester
- Lying flat on her back after the first trimester
- Smoking, including secondhand smoke
- Consuming recreational drugs and alcohol
- Cleaning up dog and cat feces
- Shampooing or touching pets bathed in flea and tick shampoos
- Consuming over-the-counter medications not recommended by her doctor
- Inhaling fumes and solvents, including hair spray and cleaning solutions
- X-rays, unless approved by her physician
- Stuffy rooms, including stuffy exercise classes
- Contact with sick children, teachers or child-care providers

Appendix Five:
Quick Protein Smoothie

An easy breakfast that's also great for alleviating morning sickness and symptoms of low blood sugar.

> 2 cups of blueberries, strawberries or raspberries, fresh or frozen
>
> 1 cup of milk, soy milk or yogurt
>
> 4 dry roasted nuts, such as almonds or walnuts
>
> 2 tablespoons of protein powder (25 to 30 grams), available at your health food store
>
> 4 ice cubes

Consider adding a few teaspoons of honey or drops of stevia, a natural sweetener available at your health food store.

Combine all ingredients in a blender. Secure the lid and—while firmly holding the lid in place—blend all ingredients using the low setting. Blend for 30 seconds on low, then 10 seconds on high. Serve with a straw.

Appendix Six:
Easy Vegetable Soup

A quick snack and a great way to increase vegetable consumption. Vegetables can be replaced with other vegetables in season.

> 1 tablespoon of olive or canola oil
>
> 1 small onion, roughly diced
>
> 3 to 4 cloves of garlic, peeled and roughly diced
>
> 1 teaspoon each of fresh dill and parsley,
>   or half the amount of dried
>
> 4 cups of chicken or vegetable stock, preferably homemade
>   (i.e., not powdered or canned)
>
> 1 cup of roughly diced red or green cabbage
>
> 1 cup of roughly diced cauliflower
>
> 1 cup of green peas, fresh or frozen
>
> 1 cup of seeded and roughly diced red or yellow
>   bell peppers
>
> 1 cup of roughly diced squash or zucchini
>
> Sea salt and pepper

Using a medium flame, set a soup pot on the stovetop. After 1 minute add the olive or canola oil to the pot. After another minute, add the onion, garlic, dill and parsley. Sauté this mixture for 5 minutes, or until the onion becomes translucent. Add the chicken or vegetable broth, and increase the flame to high until the liquid boils. Add all vegetables. When the soup liquid boils again, reduce the heat to low, cover loosely with a lid and allow the soup to simmer for one hour. After one hour, add sea salt and pepper to taste and serve.

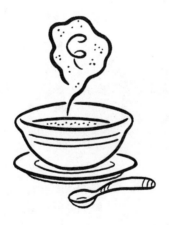

Glossary of Terms

Abruption of the placenta A life-threatening condition in which bleeding occurs behind the *placenta*.

Acid-base balance A measurement of the balance between acidity and alkalinity levels in the body (the "PH" level).

Amniotic fluid The fluid surrounding the baby.

Asymptomatic bladder infections An infection that develops without showing any of the common symptoms associated with a bladder infection.

Bacterial vaginosis An anaerobic bacterial infection in the *vagina*. When left untreated, this condition can cause premature labor, early breakage of the water and infection after the birth.

Cervical weakness A condition in which the *cervix* becomes too weak to "hold" the pregnancy, which may lead to premature delivery.

Cervix The gateway between the *vagina* and the *uterus*.

Chlamydia A microorganism, usually transmitted sexually, that may cause blindness in infants delivered vaginally when left untreated.

Doula A paid birthing coach.

Ectopic pregnancy   A pregnancy that develops outside of the *uterus*. If treatment is delayed, this condition can become life-threatening for the mother.

Edema   Water retention that causes swelling in the soft tissue of the body, especially in the hands and feet.

Electrolytes   A collection of minerals found in the body, including potassium chloride, manganese, magnesium and sodium.

Embryo   The term for a *fetus* in the very early stages pregnancy.

Epidural   A nerve pain block routinely used in delivery that is considered far safer and more effective than sedation.

Estrogen   A female hormone that the body produces more of during pregnancy.

Fasting insulin level   The measurement of the insulin hormone after an overnight fast.

Fetus   The general medical term for a baby.

Gardinella   The predominate bacteria in an infection called *bacterial vaginosis*.

Homeopathic remedies   Nonpharmaceutical health-care products sold over-the-counter that are prepared according to the natural homeopathic health-care philosophy.

Hydrocortisone cream   An over-the-counter cream applied externally to help relieve itching and eczema.

Hydrogenated oil	A saturated oil that has been heated and become harmful to the cells of the body.
In utero	A term that refers to something that happens in the mother's uterus.
Kick Journal	A journal in which the mother records the daily "kicks" or movements of the baby, twice daily for 20 to 30 minutes.
Lactobacillus acidophilus	The "friendly" bacteria in the intestinal tract and *vagina.*
Lymphatic blood flow	The flow of blood through the lymphatic system, the drainage system of the body.
Mycoplasma	An organism that causes a cervical and uterine infection.
Oligohydramnion	An abnormal decrease in the amount of *amniotic fluid.*
Perinatologist	An obstetrician and gynecologist who specializes in high-risk pregnancy and "diagnosis obstetric and genetic procedure."
Placenta	The bridge between the mother's body and the baby that implants inside the *uterus* and delivers nutrition.
Placenta previa	A condition in which the *placenta* sits directly on top of the *cervix.*
Polyhydramnion	An abnormal increase in the amount of *amniotic fluid.*

Preeclampsia A serious condition that occurs when women develop high blood pressure during pregnancy.

Progesterone A female hormone that the body produces more of during pregnancy.

Sublingual Under the tongue.

Ultrasound A procedure that produces an image of the baby on a monitor.

Umbilical cord An internal cord that connects the baby to the *placenta*.

Ureter The tube that connects that kidneys to the bladder.

Uterus The internal organ where the fertilized egg implants and the baby develops.

Vagina The internal portion of the female genitalia.

Vaginal beta strep An abnormal growth of beta strep bacteria in the *vagina*. When left untreated, this condition can lead to a fatal infection in some infants.

Vulva The external portion of the female genitalia, often mistakenly called the *vagina*. The vulva includes the lips, or labia.

Index

A

abdominal workouts, 76
acetaminophen, 122
acid-base balance, 20, 73
acidic stomach, 124–125
acid reflux, 124–125
acrylic nails, 117
activities. *see* exercise
acupressure bracelets, 19
acupuncture, 48, 76, 99
additives, 128, 197
adrenal deficiency, 158
aerobics, 84
African Americans, 194
aged cheese, 138
alcohol, 27, 198
allergic sensitivity, 136
allergist, 21
alpha lipoic acid, 158
amniocentesis, 195
amniotic fluid, 145–147
anemia, 74
ankles, swollen, 94–97
antacids, 124
antibiotics, 132
antihistamines, 51
antiperspirants, 38
apples, 154
appointments
  see doctor's appointments
arnica, 165
artificial colors, 23, 197
artificial sweeteners, 23
Ashkenazi Jews, 194
asymptomatic bacteriuria, 131
athletics. *see* exercise

B

baby's growth rate.
  see growth rate of baby
back pain, 76–77, 135
back support belts, 77

bacterial infection, 110
bacterial vaginosis, 136
bad moods, 44
baths, 38
B complex vitamin, 45
beans, 154, 155
beauty products, 115–116
beauty treatments, 117–118
bed rest, 89–91, 159
beer. *see* alcohol
belching, 126–127
berries, 154
betaine, 126
beta strep, vaginal, 137, 138
big breasts. *see* breasts
bike riding, 84
bikini waxing, 117
birthing centers, 181, 183
birthing classes, 58, 185
birthing plan, 186
bladder culture, 132, 196
bladder infections, 131–133, 196
bladder infection test, 177
bleaching hair, 117
bleeding, vaginal, 77, 110, 164–167
blood pressure, 46
blood tests, 193
blood volume, 72
blurred vision, 47, 97, 161
body type, 32
body waxing, 117
body wraps, 118
bras, 38
Braxton Hicks contractions, 172
bread, 25, 138, 154, 155
breasts
    enlargement of, 38–39
    nipples of, 39, 40–41
    size of, 41
    tenderness of, 38–39
breath, shortness of, 47, 135
burping, *see* belching
butter, 25, 155

C

caffeine, 27, 197
cakes, 155
calcium supplements, 78, 172
calling doctor.
  see doctor, when to call
candy, 155
canned food, 26
canola oil, 25, 155
carbohydrates, 25, 47, 138, 155
cardiologist, 80
carpal tunnel syndrome, 98–100
carrots, 155
cats, 119, 198
cereal, 154, 155
cervical weakness, 178–179
cesarean section, 57, 151, 181, 186
cheese, 138, 154
cherries, 154
children, lifting, 88
chiropractic manipulations, 48, 76
chlamydia, 137
chocolate, 197
chocolate milk, 50
Chorionic villi sampling (CVS), 193
chromium picolinate, 156, 158
chromosomal defects, 193
cilantro, 95
classes, birthing, 58, 185
cleaning solutions, 198
coaching at delivery, 64–66
cocoa, 27, 50, 197
Coenzyme Q-10, 160
coffee, 27, 197
cold feet, 162
cold hands, 162
cold medications, 50
colds, 122–123
cologne, 21
colostrum cream, 138
colostrum extract, 123
constipation, 101, 103–105
contractions, 83, 175–177
cookies, 155
corn, 155

crackers, 25, 154, 155
cramping, 110
cranberries, 132
cravings, 33
crying, 45
C-section. *see* cesarean section
CT scans, 76
cucumber, 95, 161

D

dairy, 24, 26, 154
decaffeinated coffee, 27
decreased amniotic fluid, 145–147
deep-fried foods, 26
deep penetration, 108
dehydration, 46, 72, 83, 128
delivery
  fears about, 57–58, 64–66
  locations for, 180–183
  options for, 184–186
deodorant, 21, 38
depression, 45, 69–70
DES, 178
desserts, 27
DHA fish oil capsules, 155
diabetes of pregnancy, 153–156
diarrhea, 78, 112, 127, 128
  magnesium supplements and, 49,
    78, 95
diet
  baby's growth and, 148
  constipation and, 103
  fast baby growth and, 151
  food shopping and, 21, 32
  foods to avoid in, 197
  headaches and, 49
  hypoglycemia and, 157
  ideal, 23–28
  indigestion and, 125
  morning sickness and, 18–19
  organic food and, 21
  preeclampsia and, 159
  sensitivity to smell and, 21
  showing interest in, 60, 63
  snacks and, 45, 157
  weight gain and, 33–34

X

X-rays, 76, 198

Y

yeast infections, 136, 138
yellow discharge, 137
yellow skin, 162
yoga, 85, 111
yokes, of eggs, 26

Z

zinc, 123
Zoloft, 50